RELATIONAL CARE

Relational Care focuses on how people working in and around healthcare can improve the delivery of whole person care. This text integrates Systems Theory and a range of communication tools to support readers in working collaboratively and developing individualized road maps for difficult conversations.

Focusing on the relationships between patient, family, and clinician, known as the Relational System, the authors explore how effective communication in healthcare can improve the well-being of all. Beginning with theoretical chapters, the Personal System is described as body, mind, and spirit. Using both Systems encourages readers to see the whole person as they practice. The book incorporates how relational practice improves care in topics such as grief, end-of-life care, stress, and burnout, giving bad news and resolving conflict. Each chapter includes case studies, reflective questions, and prompts for critical thinking to help the reader embed their learning.

This practice changing textbook will be useful to a range of health practitioners, including nurses, Physician Assistants, physicians, and more. It can be used as a supplemental reading for medical interviewing and communications courses

Lisa Zammit taught as an assistant professor at South University for over 10 years, teaching surgery, bioethics, and geriatrics. With degrees in Surgeon Assistant and Physician Assistant studies, she worked in a variety of clinical settings. Her clinical experience included critical care, surgery, emergency medicine, and research. While in Savannah, she served on the regional hospital's medical ethics board. While obtaining her Master's in Health Science at George Washington University, she focused on communication issues with Patients and Families, particularly End-of-Life conversations. During this time, she began collaboration with Georgeanne Schopp who informally supervised Lisa's Master's submission.

Georgeanne Schopp obtained her Master's Degree in Family and Child Development. While practicing as a Marriage and Family Therapist, she specialized in Thanatology and Grief. She supervised psychotherapy students, novices, and medical and mental health clinicians. Her experience in training medical professionals, clergy, and the public in care of the ill, dying, and bereaved was instrumental in the development of Relational Care.

Utilizing their extensive clinical, teaching, and research experiences, the authors bring a unique and valuable perspective to the Patient/Family/Clinician relationship. Authoring two publications on communication issues, the partners teach *Telling Bad News* and *Systems Theory in Relational Care* to PA students and professionals, MDs, mental health professionals, and nurse practitioners. The collaboration of these two disciplines – medicine and psychotherapy – culminates in Relational Care.

RELATIONAL CARE

Improving Communication in
Healthcare

Lisa Zammit and Georgeanne Schopp

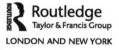
Routledge
Taylor & Francis Group

LONDON AND NEW YORK

Cover image: © Getty Images

First published 2022
by Routledge
2 Park Square, Milton Park, Abingdon, Oxon OX14 4RN

and by Routledge
605 Third Avenue, New York, NY 10158

Routledge is an imprint of the Taylor & Francis Group, an informa business

British Library Cataloguing-in-Publication Data
A catalogue record for this book is available from the British Library

Library of Congress Cataloging-in-Publication Data
Names: Zammit, Lisa, author. | Schopp, Georgeanne, author.
Title: Relational care : improving communication in healthcare / Lisa
    Zammit, Georgeanne Schopp.
Description: Milton Park, Abingdon, Oxon ; New York, NY : Routledge,
    2022. | Includes bibliographical references and index.
Identifiers: LCCN 2021058331 (print) | LCCN 2021058332 (ebook) |
    ISBN 9781032189833 (hardback) | ISBN 9781032189826 (paperback) |
    ISBN 9781003257219 (ebook)
Subjects: LCSH: Medical care. | Health services administration. | Health
    planning. | Communication in medicine.
Classification: LCC RA393 .Z36 2022 (print) | LCC RA393 (ebook) |
    DDC 362.1068—dc23/eng/20211208
LC record available at https://lccn.loc.gov/2021058331
LC ebook record available at https://lccn.loc.gov/2021058332

ISBN: 978-1-032-18983-3 (hbk)
ISBN: 978-1-032-18982-6 (pbk)
ISBN: 978-1-003-25721-9 (ebk)

DOI: 10.4324/9781003257219

Typeset in Bembo
by Apex CoVantage, LLC

To our families who care for us, our colleagues who encourage us, our patients who teach us, and our students who lead us.

CONTENTS

FIGURES

TABLES

BOXES

PREFACE

This book has been a compelling journey. We met in desperation, when Lisa was tasked with telling her hospitalized patients they were going to die. Seeking help and/or training, her minister referred her to Georgeanne. Trained as a therapist and thanatologist, Georgeanne provided guidance and insight. It altered Lisa's classic medical training and patient care.

Georgeanne and Lisa developed a supervisory relationship for her Master's work. That resulted in their first publication, *Breaking Bad News: Communication Skills for Difficult Conversations*. The partners began teaching and writing regularly. With a lifetime of personal and professional experiences for the authors, the classroom is where Relational Care emerged and developed.

Each chapter may be used independently and begins with objectives. *Italicized* case studies emphasize and illustrate difficult concepts. Based on actual cases, identities are changed to maintain anonymity. At the end of each chapter, Questions for Reflection provoke personal thinking. There are no "correct" answers. The intent is to stimulate reflection, learning, debate, and research. Appendices provide additional resources and role play scenarios for practice.

This book is organized into four parts:

Part I: **Opening Our Eyes** This section establishes the foundational concept of Relational Care. It defines and describes components that create a working vocabulary for the text. "Personhood," including Body, Mind, and Spirit, and the "Healthcare Collaboration," including Patient, Family, and Clinician, are systemically and visually explored. The problem of poor compliance and Patient dissatisfaction is elaborated. The fracturing of healthcare is discussed and explained in the light of Relational Care.

Part II: **Elements of the Whole** The elements of Body, Mind, and Spirit, known as the Personal System, are addressed through the "lenses" of

Relational Care. The elements of Relational System are comprised of the Patient, Family, and Clinician.

Part III: Barriers and Baggage This section deals with threats to good communication and Healthcare Collaboration. Grief, special populations, dying and death, stress, compassion fatigue, and burnout are described and discussed. Recognizing, preventing, or avoiding these issues protects and cares for Patient, Family, and Clinician.

Part IV: Creating Solutions Tools and skills are included in this section. Improved communication and self-care is promoted and encouraged for all healthcare providers. Clear communication and conflict resolution "bridges the gap" in difficult and emotional conversations.

ACKNOWLEDGMENTS

There was no lengthy discussion about whether this book needed to be written. It was a journey we were *called* to make. In the process of writing, the authors discovered how much better the writing and ideas flowed when working together. Clinical practice, teaching, researching, and writing together, synergistically developed the concepts of Relational Care. We are grateful for God's inspiration.

The authors recognize support throughout this process. Margie Carson was our initial grammatical editor who educated us on the subtleties of writing. Theresa Morris offered her retreat and support for uninterrupted production. Valerie Yaughn, with her library expertise, assisted us with research at South University, Savannah. Amy Vandenbroucke provided invaluable input regarding POLST. Ed Towey, with Aging With Dignity, was generous in granting us access to *Five Wishes*.

Our initial readers, Dr. Julia Mikell, Rev. Robert Townsend, Dr. Robert DiBenedetto, Dr. Katherine Klock-Powell, and Rosemary Allen clarified our focus with their feedback. Thank you for giving us your time and attention! To the Taylor and Francis team, Grace McInnes and Evie Lonsdale (et al.), who recognized the vision of Relation Care, we appreciate your taking us through the publication process.

No book gets written without the support, patience, and generosity of spirit from family and friends. How blessed we are for your presence in our lives.

To all those who inspired us by their struggles and joys – clients, teachers, mentors, colleagues, classmates, students, and most of all to the Patients, Families, and Clinicians for following the *call*. We are honored by our journey together.

GLOSSARY

Acute Physiology, Age, Chronic Health Evaluation (APACHE III): A clinical prognostication tool used to provide initial risk stratification for severely ill patients and provide risk estimates for hospital mortality in individual ICU patients.

Adaptation: The change or process of change as the person becomes accustomed to a new situation.

Advance Directives (AD): A legal document describing the medical care the patient wishes to receive or not, should they become unable to communicate with family or healthcare providers. An AD typically will designate one or more persons with Medical Durable Power of Attorney to make decisions on the patient's behalf.

Allow Natural Death (AND): An alternative order to Do Not Resuscitate; AND is a plan that emphasizes comfort care as opposed to withdrawal of curative or life-sustaining care.

Boundaries: Limits and borders to personal space and obligations define boundaries. Expressing boundaries includes asserting personal values, rules, and limits within relationships.

Comorbidity: The presence of one or more disease processes in addition to the primary or presenting complaint/disease. Comorbidities impact the primary disease and/or influence the care plan.

Congruence: The synchronicity of body language with oral communication.

Countertransference: A redirection of a clinician's feelings toward a patient, based on unrelated interactions.

Curative Care: Interventions with the primary purpose of achieving a cure, returning to baseline health, stabilizing a disease process, or bringing a meaningful and measurable improvement in the health status of the patient.

Dementia: A group of conditions characterized by impairment of at least two brain functions, such as memory loss and judgment.

Distress: Abnormal levels of stress, which, if prolonged, can lead to compassion fatigue and burnout.

Empathy: Understanding another's thoughts and feelings from their point of view.

Eustress: Normal stress, generally experienced as normal or beneficial to the individual. Eustress generates excitement, creativity, meaning, fulfillment, and satisfaction.

Family Dynamics: The patterns of interactions among members of a family unit and the factors that influence the interactions and individual behaviors.

Hospice: End-of-Life care provided by a team of health professionals, mental health professionals, and spiritual leaders, a multidisciplinary approach emphasizing the comfort and care of the dying patient. Although aggressive medical therapy is available, it is for comfort purposes only, not curative. Hospice care not only provides services to the patient but also supports the family, with grief counseling.

Incongruence: Inappropriate effect, or when one's behavior or evaluation of a situation does not match reality.

Intensive Care Unit (ICU): ICU care provides more aggressive medical care. With specialized technology and available immediate response, specialized ICUs include Cardiac, Medical, Med/Surg, Neonatal, Neurology, Pediatric, and others.

Living Will: Replaced by Advance Directives, a Living Will is a written document describing interventions a patient does or does not want to be done on their behalf in a medical crisis. Although rare, a Living Will remains a legal document.

Medical Durable Power of Attorney (MDPOA): A person designated by the patient to make medical care decisions on the patient's behalf. MDPOA goes into effect should the patient become unable to communicate or decide for themselves. The designee has the legal right to make decisions and is authorized to do so in the patient's Advance Directives. Most often a family member (spouse, child, sibling), the MDPOA can be anyone the patient designates.

Memory: The process of encoding and storing data and its retrieval.

Mirroring: The conscious or unconscious behavior of imitating the gesture, speech, and body language of another person as a form of empathy and presence.

Moral Injury: Moral injury is a trauma characterized by guilt, existential crisis, and loss of trust that is developed after a perceived moral violation. In healthcare, moral injury most often occurs when Clinicians are prevented, by either scarcity or administrative restrictions, from delivering the care needed to their Patients.

Morbidity: A disease state or symptom. Morbidity does not necessarily mean mortality (or death) although it can contribute to demise.

Multidisciplinary Team (MDT): A team of specialists from various fields of practice to integrate and coordinate care of the patient. Various disciplines include, but are not limited to, medical specialties, mental health care, spiritual leaders, and therapists (speech, occupational, physical, respiratory, etc.).

Palliative Care: Palliative Care emphasizes relief of symptoms versus curative care. Although associated with hospice care, patients can receive palliative care at any time during the course of their disease. For example, a cancer patient may continue to receive chemotherapy in palliative care. Timing or dosage may be altered to alleviate the side effects of therapy. Although curative treatment can still be given in palliative care, it is no longer the primary goal.

Patient's Rights: The legal and ethical issues in the provider–patient relationship include a person's right to privacy, the right to quality medical care without prejudice, the right to make informed decisions about care and treatment options, and the right to refuse treatment.

Personhood: Elements of self, Personhood is composed of the intersection of Body, Mind, and Spirit.

Physician Orders for Life-Sustaining Treatment (POLST): An order set based upon the patient's Advance Directives. These medical orders delineate therapy and preferences that can be applied in any medical setting, including hospital and doctor's offices.

Post-Traumatic Stress Disorder (PTSD): A mental health disorder triggered by a severe traumatic event. Symptoms include re-experiencing the event; avoidance of memories, thoughts, and feelings of the event; negative cognition and mood; and arousal marked by aggressive, reckless, or self-destructive behaviors including sleep disturbances and hypervigilance.

Presence: The act of being present is eliminating the distraction (also known as "noise") of outside influences and focusing on the here and now of what is happening, to the exclusion of everything else.

Reductionism: The belief that understanding complex issues can be mastered by breaking them down into simple, basic mechanisms.

Reframing: A shift in mindset, enabling viewing a situation, person, or relationship from a different perspective.

Resilience: The ability to adapt in the face of adversity, trauma, tragedy, or other significant stressors.

Secondary Gain: An advantage that occurs secondary to stated or real illness. This can include using illness for personal advantage. It is demonstrated by exaggerating symptoms, consciously using symptoms for gain (attention or monetary), and unconsciously presenting symptoms with no physiological basis.

Secondary Traumatic Stress Disorder (STSD): Emotional distress that results when an individual hears first hand or witnesses another's traumatic event.

Sequential Organ Failure Assessment Score (SOFA): A clinical assessment tool used to predict ICU mortality based on lab results and clinical data.

Situational Depression: A normal reaction to a stressful event. Situational depression is a personal response to what instigates the depression. As opposed to clinical Depression, it is not a Mood Disorder. Typically, situational depression resolves in a timely manner and does not require medication.

Stages of Malignancy: Staging is a nomenclature used to describe the severity and spread of the patient's malignancy. Although there are other staging nomenclatures for specific cancers, the general system uses a TNM system. Based on the size of the tumor (T), the spread of the cancer to regional lymph nodes (N), and the sites of distant metastasis, spread, in other organs (M), TNM staging is used to determine the patient's overall staging as Stage 0, I, II, III, or IV.

Stress: The physical and emotional response to demand. Stress can be normal, also known as eustress, or excessive, which can lead to mental and physical health side effects.

Sympathy: The feeling of pity and sorrow for someone else's misfortune.

Vicarious Traumatization: The negative reaction to trauma exposure while serving victims of trauma.

PART I
Opening Our Eyes

1

INTRODUCTION

Every day brings new advances leading to countless "medical miracles." Historically, these were seen as an act of God. Today, technology delivers "miracles" on a daily basis.

As practitioners, competence increases with continuing education, improved technology, and innovative treatment options. Medicine has progressed far beyond the "rational medicine" of Hippocrates. The personal relationship between the patient and the clinician has evolved. The impersonal third party, technology, now dominates.

Historically, medical care was provided by members of the family and community. There was no differentiation of physical, mental, and spiritual care. As knowledge and learning expanded through universities, there was a philosophical shift in caregiving. By the 17th century, Rene Descarte's Reductionist Theory promoted the separation of care of body and soul. He also introduced the third component, the mind, as an additional entity of the whole person (Lewis, 2007). Reductionism, the study of the body, mind, and spirit as distinct disciplines, resulted in the isolation of care seen today.

The advent of Cartesian philosophy signaled a change in the caregivers' approach to the patient disease process. Opposed to the previous concept of a person in need of care, solace, and salvation in their final hours, the patient became an object of study. As our knowledge base advanced, experts in medical, mental, or spiritual care concentrated exclusively on their focus of study.

How clinicians perceive relationships with patients originated from End-of-Life care and the hospice movement. Addressing the physical suffering of the dying patient is inadequate. Providing an integrated approach to care for patient and family members' mental, physical, and spiritual suffering results in healing. Originally limited to caring for the dying, the consequences of change are far-reaching. How clinicians communicate impacts every patient, not just the acutely ill or dying.

DOI: 10.4324/9781003257219-2

Despite advances, patient and family satisfaction in care has diminished (Lewis, 2007). This inverse relationship has taken generations to develop and decades to recognize. Unless patients are viewed as much more than diagnoses and/or treatment protocols, the *whole* patient is not cared for. Although attempts have been made to improve patient communication and satisfaction, education on this topic is limited to a chapter in a textbook or a class under the heading of mental health or ethics (Berg et al., 2013). The esoteric classroom discussion does not integrate easily into clinical practice. As a result, quality of care languishes. Clinicians become frustrated and burned out.

Relational Care creates more than a partnership. It is collaboration. Its value lies in establishing and maintaining communication among patient, family, and clinician. "No man is an island" is more than a quote from John Donne. It describes the necessity of seeing each patient as a person in relationship with the clinician, their disease, and their world. Practitioners are trained to look at specifics of the disease process – the pathophysiology. Relational Care techniques determine causation of the patient's symptoms as well as the impact of the disease.

Two patients with the same dataset illustrate how Relational Care works. A 20-year-old white male presents with a 4-day history of cough, fever, and productive sputum. In Relational Care, the curious provider engages the patient in conversation. He works a 40-hour week, tending bar on the weekends to pay for graduate school, which he attends during the day. To stay awake and functional on an average of 4 hours of sleep a night, the patient has resorted to multiple energy drinks. A different perspective emerges which may or may not require more than medical intervention.

The same clinical presentation in a 20-year-old female may yield a different relational story. In conversation, she reveals she has dropped out of college. She works as a waitress to support her increasing methamphetamine habit. Her family has thrown her out of the house, and she has been forced to move in with her boyfriend. After talking for a few minutes, the patient also admits that she has had numerous sexual contacts while under the influence. She has lost substantial weight in the past 3 months.

With Relational Care, the patient, as a person with different values and social factors in place, adds to the simple pathophysiology of the presentation. Both cases present with the same symptoms – a case of pneumonia. Without knowledge of their lifestyles, standard evidence-based treatment would be prescribed. Relational Care reveals a more accurate "picture" of each patient. Their family and social environment suggest targeted treatment options and control of risk factors. Discovery is made during a relational conversation, not during a standard clinical evaluation.

The definition of health is complete physical, mental, and spiritual well-being (Lewis, 2007). This definition, authored by the World Health Organization, recognizes three integral parts of **Personhood** – Body, Mind, and Spirit. Personhood is determined by the integration of these three elements. In addition to this holistic relationship, the **Healthcare Collaboration** comprises the Patient, Family, and Clinician. Just as Body, Mind, and Spirit impact and influence each other, so does the relationship among Patient, Family, and Clinician. This use of Systems Theory expands healthcare.

Ignoring any element of the person or the healthcare relationship may cause suffering. Imbalance is created, even in an otherwise physically healthy person. As a practitioner, our avenues for healing are greatly increased when we pay attention to the relationships that are present in the physical, intellectual/emotional, and spiritual elements. Relational Care offers healing potential that moves beyond technology. As opposed to treating pathophysiology alone, awareness of the whole person in patient care expands our options and increases effectiveness in healing.

Relational Care does not take the place of understanding bioethics. Nor does it consist of new mental health interventions. Relational Care is a way of seeing the Patient through different lenses. It integrates the whole person into the disease process that Clinicians are trained identify and treat. Relational Care recognizes the value and effectiveness in addressing all aspects of relationships among Patient, Family, and Clinicians. The purpose of this text is to educate Clinicians on the possibilities of integrated Relational Care. Additionally, it provides self-protection and self-care concepts to remain effective and healthy.

Relational Care is personal. It changes how we communicate with our own Families, how we process disease and death, and how we care for ourselves and each other. It becomes part of what we are. It makes us better human beings and practitioners. Envisioning the Patient and the Clinician–Patient relationship adds depth to care and improves Patient satisfaction and compliance.

In 1996, the Joint Commission on Accreditation of Healthcare Organizations (JCAHO) issued a policy requiring hospitals to provide pastoral counseling. In 1998, the Association of American Medical Colleges responded with the Medical School Objectives Project where coursework was required connecting spirituality and health (Puchalski, 2006). In 2004, JCAHO published a Spiritual Assessment Question guide (Appendix B.1). This series of suggested questions was recommended as an additional assessment tool.

Patients have significant concerns and questions regarding their spirituality and terminal condition. Despite that, less than 20% were able to discuss these issues with their providers (Mahler et al., 2010). Conversations, in *relationship*, should not be limited to Patient and physician. Family, other caregivers, and other Clinicians need to be included. The willingness to begin these conversations and recognizing appropriate timing are critical skills. Patients expect Clinicians to initiate these conversations.

Establishing a relationship requires time to develop and evolve. Patients want their values and needs appreciated and included in their care plan (Ellis & Campbell, 2004). Families want help in knowing how to care for their loved ones. Fears and personal needs require acknowledgment and support (Nelson, 2005).

Working with chronically and critically ill Patients is physically, mentally, and spiritually exhausting. Maintaining a healthy balance is vital. Relational Care offers resources and tools to prevent compassion fatigue and burnout.

Case studies have been included and appear in italicized text boxes. Some of the cases have no clear resolution. Some seem miraculous. These cases were chosen not to demonstrate a standard protocol or "sure fire fix." They demonstrate how openness to Patient and Family concerns and awareness of outside influences impact care and decision-making. There is no standardized protocol that, once learned, can be employed in every situation. Relational Care is a personal relationship in caregiving encompassing all members of the Healthcare Collaboration.

Questions for Reflection

1   Consider your typical Patient/Clinician interaction. What part does Family play in the Patient's decisions regarding care?
2   Electronic Medical Records improve the accuracy and efficiency of medical documentation. How have they influenced your Patient/Clinician relationship?

References

Berg, G., Whitney, M., Wentlin, C., Hervey, A., & Nyberg, S. (2013). Physician assistant program education on spirituality and religion in patient encounters. *Journal of Physician Assistant Education, 24*(2), 24–27. https://doi.org/10/1097/01367895-201324020-00006

Ellis, M., & Campbell, J. (2004). Patients' views about discussing spiritual issues with primary care physicians. *Southern Medical Journal, 97*(12), 1158–1164. https://doi.org/10.1097/01.DMJ.0000146486.69217.EE

Lewis, M. (2007). *Medicine and care of the dying* (p. 34). Oxford University Press.

Mahler, D., Selecky, P., Harrod, C., Hansen-Flaschen, J., O'Donnell, D., & Waller, A. (2010). American College of Chest Physicians consensus statement on the management of dyspnea in patients with advanced lung or heart disease. *Chest Journal, 137*(3), 674–691. https://doi.org/10.1378/chest.09-1543

Nelson, R. (2005). The compassionate clinician: Attending to the spiritual needs of self and others. *Critical Care Medicine, 33*(12), 2841–2842.

Puchalski, C. (2006). *A time for listening and caring* (pp. 22–25). Oxford University Press.

2

DEFINING THE PROBLEM

Objectives

1   Describe and understand the application of Systems Theory in medicine
2   Define and describe the Personal System and Relational System
3   Describe Relational Care and its components

Introduction

Medical training relies on formulas based on the science of the Body. The total person is not supported by this framework which treats Body, Mind, or Spirit, as specialization silos. Ignoring care of one aspect of Personhood creates an unhealthy balance. Bernie Siegel (1998) posits this imbalance as a source of modern man's unhappiness and sense of unfulfillment. Siegel (1998), Kaplan (2014), and Keck (1993), a surgeon, a psychotherapist, and a minister, suggest this may be the basis for many illnesses and/or treatment failures.

Fracturing of care means the Patient does not regularly see the same practitioner. Today's mega-practices do not foster relationship between Patient and Clinician. The Clinician's knowledge of the Patient is generated from a quick scanning of the chart. The empiric methodology of electronic medical records exacerbates this impersonal, generic care. Practitioner's time with the Patient is limited. Reimbursement issues shrink available time further.

The number of comorbidities and complex diagnoses increases the number of Clinicians involved in care. Many multidisciplinary teams (MDT) exist in name only. MDTs are "Patient oriented" but usually exclude the Patient in team meetings. Family is never incorporated into care.

Clinicians practice autonomously, with each focused on their specific specialty (O'Daniel & Rosenstein, 2008). The Joint Commission on Accreditation of

DOI: 10.4324/9781003257219-3

Healthcare Organization (2005) cites communication failures as the leading cause of medication errors, delay in treatments, and wrong site surgeries. With poor communication, patient safety is at risk.

Isolation of Patient and Clinician interferes with relationship building. Patients and Families have little information regarding the disease, much less a relationship with their Clinicians. In times of crisis, the Clinician becomes the default decision-maker. Necessary data for difficult decisions are missing without established relationships.

Systems Theory

A basic understanding of Systems Theory provides additional lenses for clinical practice. It visualizes and organizes data and operations, emphasizing connections. Systems Theory allows Clinicians to see possibilities outside of the physical care of their Patients. It focuses on the relationships among all elements rather than the isolation of each one. Systems Theory illustrates how a change in one affects a change in all. A geared mechanism, for example, an analog watch, is the classic description of how Systems work. When one gear moves, all other gears must also move. The rate, degree, and direction of each movement will differ.

Relational Care merges Systems Theory with healthcare. It is more than a treatment paradigm or protocol – it recognizes the Patient as a gear in relationship with

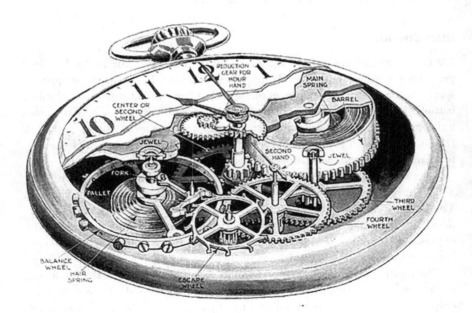

FIGURE 2.1 Internal components of an analog watch. Each gear interacts with others, all moving at different rates and/or directions.

Source: Seielstad (2022)

others. Relational Care elevates the Personhood of the Patient in addition to the disease and clinical caregiving. It values the importance of the Patient, Family, and Clinician IN RELATIONSHIP. Just as the nuclear "blood family" includes friendships, Clinicians include the entire care team. Relational Care goes beyond the medical and legal standards of Informed Consent. It encompasses the medical knowledge, ethics, personal values, and preferences of each member of the Healthcare Collaboration.

Body

The anatomy and physiology of the Body are well known, unlike the Mind and Spirit. It is far easier to describe, evaluate, and treat the physical body. Based on scientific process, the Body is the Clinician's "comfort zone." As complex as it is, the body is the most understood and documented aspect of self.

Linear processes in medicine reduce patient care to diagnose the disease, begin treatment, reduce symptoms, and cure the problem. The specialist practice narrows this focus even more. Clinicians see the patient as a diseased organ system: the cardiovascular, pulmonary, gastrointestinal, etc. Focusing attention on a specific organ limits vision and neglects care of other components of the person. The language and vocabulary of the medical professional are both exclusive and exclusionary.

Mind

The brain is the physiological and anatomical structure of the Mind. What and how we think illustrates the brain working as it gathers data, interprets it, reasons, remembers, and imagines. The Body gathers data through the senses. The Mind processes the data and rationalizes the experience. Intellect reasons and understands. Interpretation of events is subsequently stored in long-term memory.

Memory is the warehouse function of the Mind, while perception is the interpretative function. What is stored and what is remembered contributes to that person's reality. Perception interprets memory which is altered with time and new information.

BOX 2.1 HEATHER

Heather presented to her primary care provider with general malaise, loss of energy, distractibility, and poor sleep. In her therapy referral, she demonstrated appropriate intellect, insight, and judgment. Heather reported no suicidal or homicidal ideation.

> *Heather, age 51, was always considered the "baby" of the family, even though she had a twin brother born only 10 minutes before her. As an elite educator, she was regarded as a model of competency in her field.*

> *Heather's perception of herself supported the family myth of incompe-*
> *tence because she was the youngest . . . and female. Despite a successful*
> *career and loving family, Heather was depressed.*
>
> *In therapeutic session, she was asked to recount her favorite childhood*
> *memory. Heather told the story of sitting on her grandfather's knee as he*
> *read to her and her twin. When the therapist observed that Heather had*
> *equal status in her grandfather's eyes, she smiled through her tears. Her*
> *perspective of being the "baby" which translated into "not good enough"*
> *had forever changed.*
>
> A memory may have filters that allow influences on what actually happened.
> Heather believed she was "less than" her brother. Recalling her favorite mem-
> ory in the therapeutic setting changed her perception by paying attention to
> the details of the memory. She and her brother were equally loved by their
> grandfather. Heather was indeed "good enough."

Heather's depression was rooted in the core of the family myth. Being female and the "baby," her competency and successes were never recognized. Returning to her childhood memory, Heather was able to debunk her lifelong perception. She could accept herself for what she **is** – a competent, capable, successful person despite the family myth.

Spirit

Spirit is personally defined with no physical boundaries. Composed of the value system and influenced by emotion, one's character or soul is developed. Morals and values are "housed" in this amorphous entity. The Mind influences and articulates the Spirit.

Emotions are the expression in a nonthinking, non–planning process that directs behavior. In other words, we can be sad about a loss without consciously thinking about it. The Spirit triggers the Mind to recall a memory. The memory refreshes the emotional response of the Spirit, positive or negative.

The interplay among the Body, Mind, and Spirit reflects the holistic system. Each element influences the other and is repeated in interactions. The relationship among Body, Mind, and Spirit is augmented and expanded in relationships among Patient, Family, and Clinician. When these are recognized, explored, and valued, clear communication and consensus develops.

Attempts at care of the whole person exist. Complementary and Alternative Medicine is known by the acronym CAM, or by the term "holistic medicine." Holistic health philosophy focuses on the importance of treating Body, Mind, *and* Spirit. Most CAM therapies are unavailable in US hospitals. Typically, CAM practices house more than one specialist. Practice members include medical clinicians in care of the Body, mental health practitioners in care of the Mind, and religious professionals in care of the Spirit (Kaplan, 2014). Each clinician is aware of the capabilities and referral parameters of their colleagues.

Osteopathy, once considered a form of CAM, is now accepted as conventional medical practice. CAM therapies include herbal medicine, acupuncture, massage, chiropractic therapy, etc. Schools that train in holistic medicine with comprehensive care of Body, Mind, *and* Spirit are limited in number. This training does not easily foster specialization such as cardiology, surgery, neurology, etc. While holistic care focuses on the whole person, the relationships among Patient, Family, and Clinician are neglected.

Integration of behavioral sciences into standard medical care faces substantial challenges. Difficulties include lack of training models, inexperience with multiple disciplines, appointment time constraints, and insurance reimbursement. Despite success in limited trials and federal mandates for concurrent psychological and medical care, implementation in current practice is rare (Funk et al., 2008).

Family Dynamics

Each one of us lives in a different and unique family. A family of four consists of two parents, a boy, and a girl. The father is part of a family consisting of a wife and two children; the mother's family consists of a husband and two children, etc.

Birth order, history, and roles are developed as these different "families" interact. Birth order is naturally determined unless there is fostering or adoption (formal or informal). Family history is uniquely interpreted by each individual because each person is in a different life stage, as well as a different family. Roles develop and change as families' circumstances evolve.

Maintaining equilibrium requires response to each new event. Homeostasis "maintains a state of equilibrium through feedback and communication" (Segrin & Flora, 2005, p. 33). When a family member becomes ill or suffers trauma, adaptations, for example, role shifts, reveal changes in family dynamics.

Each new circumstance is a catalyst for reactions and role changes. For example, the father, the patriarch, suffers a heart attack. The mother becomes the breadwinner. The "baby" of the family may become a designated caregiver because she is the youngest, living at home, and single. Relational Care offers insight and tools dealing with consequential changes.

Families want to be involved in their loved one's care. However, some Clinicians view family involvement as "troublemaking" or impediments to rapid treatment. Clinicians avoid communicating with families for numerous reasons. Assembling three or more parties together is difficult. Establishing a common vocabulary, mutual understanding, and cultural sensitivity may impede clear and accurate communication. Potential conflicts, overt, covert, or historical, are additional factors.

Each person is a part of many cultures including familial, ancestral, religious, regional, etc. Ignoring cultural differences and the needs of special populations creates roadblocks to successful collaboration.

Relational Care

The holistic concept of Body, Mind, and Spirit is relatively easy to understand. Integrating it into daily practice may prove to be a challenge. A visual representation of personhood illustrates how the interdependence of Body, Mind, and Spirit actually function. A simple Venn diagram of three intersecting circles illustrates how and why Relational Care is beneficial.

The relationship of the elements in Figure 2.2 intersects and overlaps, representing Personhood. Notice that the diagram allows interaction from each element with the others creating the **Personal System**. While this diagram shows each influence as equal, humans are not that simple. One individual may have more influence from the Spirit; others are more Body oriented, etc. However, the apportionment occurs; it is a dynamic blend that will shift according to events, circumstances, and experiences.

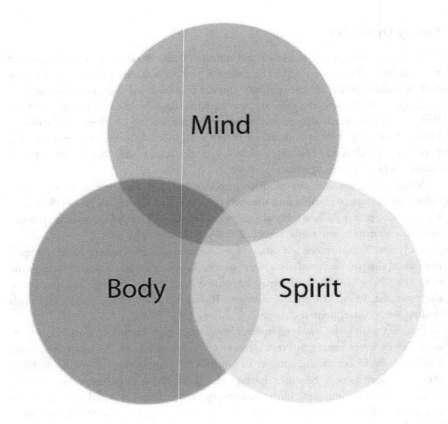

FIGURE 2.2   Body, Mind, and Spirit: the Venn diagram representing the Personal System, illustrating the interrelationship of Body, Mind, and Spirit. The intersection of all three is the "sweet spot" known as Personhood.

The health of the person is determined by the interrelationship and balance among all three elements. Even with a preponderance of one, if the other elements are being acknowledged and cared for, the total person will remain healthy. Ignoring, denying, or suppressing one element creates imbalance that adversely impacts the others.

Relational Care provides tools for visualizing changes and maintains focus on the "sweet spot." This "sweet spot" or intersection is illustrated in the Venn diagram (Figure 2.3). It depicts the Patient, Family, and Clinician interrelationship. This is called the Healthcare Collaboration.

In this **Relational System**, each element impacts and interrelates with the other. Reality is far more complex. For instance, a Patient may be medicated to relieve pain and consequently have an unclear mind. Family members may be composed of a sole significant other, a distant cousin, or a large extended family. A Clinician may be part of a multidisciplinary care team. Relationships and roles are more dynamic as the number of elements increases. It is important to appreciate the impact of individuals' Personhood (each Body, Mind, and Spirit), upon the relationships (Patient, Family, and Clinician).

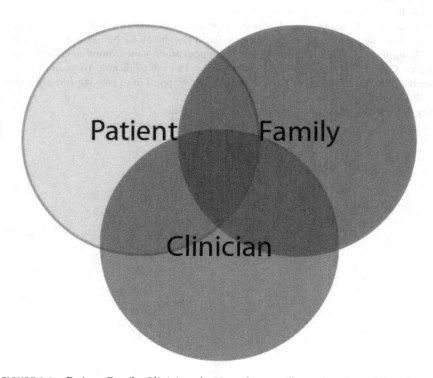

FIGURE 2.3   Patient, Family, Clinician: the Venn diagram illustrating the Relational System that includes the Patient, Family, and Clinician. The intersection of all three identifies the "sweet spot" known as the Healthcare Collaboration.

Relational Care goes beyond holistic care of Body, Mind, and Spirit, to emphasize the interrelationship of Patient, Family, and Clinician and its place in Patient care. The disease process is the common ground. It is within the confines of the disease that the Healthcare Collaboration facilitates *all* the relationships in Patient care.

Questions for Reflection

1   Using the Venn diagrams, consider your own Family. What are your roles in your Family? How have your roles changed with your increasing healthcare experience?
2   Imagine a medical emergency in your Family. Which of your roles will change?

References

Funk, M., Saraceno, B., Drew, N., & Faydi, E. (2008). Integrating mental health into primary care. *Mental Health in Family Medicine, 5*(1), 5–8.

Joint Commission on Accreditation of Healthcare Organization. (2005). *The Joint Commission guide to improving staff communication.* Joint Commission Resources.

Kaplan, G. (2014). *Total recovery.* Rodale, Inc.

Keck, R. (1993). *Sacred eyes.* Synergy Associates.

O'Daniel, M., & Rosenstein, A. (2008). *Professional communication and team collaboration.* Patient Safety and Quality: An Evidence Based Handbook for Nurses Vol 2. The Joint Commission Guide to Improving Staff Communication. Joint Commission Resources.

Segrin, C., & Flora, J. (2005). *Family communication.* Lawrence Erlbaum Association.

Seielstad, B. G. (2022). *Pocket watch.* Electronically retrieved from en.wikipedia.org/wiki/Pocketwatch

Siegel, B. (1998). *Peace, love, and healing.* Collins Publishers.

PART II

Elements of the Whole

3

BODY

Objectives

1 Define the Body
2 Discuss the similarities and differences of the terms "cure" and "heal"
3 Understand palliative care and hospice

Introduction

An understanding of the components of the Personal System and Relational System establishes common vocabulary. The elements of the whole cover Body, Mind, Spirit, and Patient, Family, Clinician.

Clinicians are caregivers. The urge to help, to "do something," is sharpened to a compulsion. When faced with serious illness or dying patients, Clinicians default to appropriate protocols for the Body. Medical training allows for rapid care in critical situations. However, focusing solely on the Body ignores the whole person.

Limited to the physiology, pathology, and treatment of bodily illness, many Clinicians never develop the skills, much less awareness, of mental or spiritual needs. The Body, with its specialized vocabulary and extensive knowledge base, is the Clinician's comfort zone. Medical communication conveys large amounts of data in a very few words. This language is intimidating and confusing to Patient and Family. It also isolates the Clinician.

Definition

The anatomical definition of the Body is the physical structure of a human being, excluding head and limbs. The body is technically limited to the trunk. Medically,

DOI: 10.4324/9781003257219-5

the body is the material of the human. It comprises the anatomical structures as well as its physiological functioning – from the corporeal to the cellular level.

A disease process is experienced by the whole Body. Although only one specific system is primarily impacted by disease or trauma, the entire Body experiences change. Accommodations and adaptations result in varying degrees. Mechanisms are brought into play to protect the Body from damage progression. White cells, angiogenesis, cortisol levels, and basic cellular metabolism accelerate in response.

The process may be sub-acute. The Patient may be unaware of pathology. However, even in the sub-acute illness or injury, microscopic scarring occurs. Cellular dysfunction occurs on multiple levels impacting tissue and/or organ systems. The result can range from undetectable cellular dysfunction to increased tissue vulnerability, organ compromise, or systemic failure.

Each insult creates a scar. It may be visible (an amputation) or microscopic (a permanently malfunctioning alveoli). Insults are cumulative, leading to the loss of health. Cellular sentience, the natural process of aging, contributes to this gradual decline.

Process

When the Body becomes symptomatic, the Patient seeks care. Occult pathology (e.g., hypertension) is revealed by routine examination even when there are no symptoms present. Clinicians understand the consequences of not treating "silent killer" diseases. Treatment prevents or delays disease progression including its impact on other systems. What is less appreciated or understood is the impact of the disease process upon Personhood.

Clinicians tend to view medicine as warfare. Cases are "won" or "lost"; the Patient lives or dies. Morbidity and mortality conferences are designed as learning opportunities. These conferences explore how to prevent or ameliorate poor outcomes. The subconscious message is "death is the enemy." As opposed to a normal biological progression of life, death is viewed as clinical error.

Treating the diagnosis according to protocol neglects the needs of the whole person. The need to cure misses the opportunities to *heal*. Within Relational Care, the Body, Mind, and Spirit are balanced allowing for restoration and healing.

Medicine focuses on recognizing signs of dying, in order to interrupt the process. Palliative care is the treatment of the Patient *without* the primary focus being cure of the disease. Rather, the goal is preserving quality of life. The Patient can receive curative medical therapy. It may be used for remediation of specific symptoms, slowing disease progression, or to obtain a specific life goal.

Curative treatment ceases when the Patient enters hospice. Symptom relief and optimizing quality of life are the primary goals. Family has the opportunity to participate in the care of the Patient. Hospice continues to educate and support the Family after the demise of their loved one. While standard care focuses solely on care of the Body, hospice attends to care of the Mind and Spirit as well.

Integration

Integrated care of Body, Mind, and Spirit has been historically limited to dying Patients. For the Patient, all three elements are integral in each decision, consciously or subconsciously. Each Patient needs freedom of choice to determine their future.

BOX 3.1   RONNIE

Personhood is a birthright; there is no minimum or maximum age requirement. Appropriate communication can reveal surprising results.

Ronnie was the middle child in a family of boys living in a neighborhood of boys. The entire family, but Ronnie in particular, was familiar with the local Emergency Department, thanks to their frequent visits. At 5 years of age, Ronnie had numerous stitches for various minor accidents.

Today's visit was prompted by a poorly aimed rock that grazed Ronnie's eyebrow. As a "frequent flyer," both Dr. Askew and Ronnie immediately recognized each other and reviewed the scars from the doctor's previous work. Dr. Askew looked at the laceration, glanced at Ronnie's mother, then looked directly at Ronnie. Negotiations began.

Ronnie very clearly and distinctly said, "I don't want that needle thing." Dr. Askew nodded. Ronnie then added, "I don't want that wrap thing either," gesturing to the papoose board hanging on the pediatric treatment room wall. Dr. Askew nodded again and replied, "You understand what that means, right?" Ronnie nodded back and said, "It will hurt and I have to hold still anyway."

To his mother's astonishment, Ron's wishes were honored and he tolerated the sutures without incident.

Both Ronnie's mother and Dr. Askew recognized and respected the 5-year-old's Personhood. In turn, Ronnie tolerated a painful procedure with fewer medications and stress. The entire Healthcare Collaboration benefited.

A terminal diagnosis allows the patient to make decisions regarding the remainder of their lives (Siegel, 1998). Each Patient establishes their own priorities. Viewed as noncompliance by Clinicians, Patient needs may trump medical protocols. Incorporating Personhood in medical therapy acknowledges Body, Spirit, and Mind.

BOX 3.2   JEANIE

Jeanie was a single 62-year-old female treated and in remission for throat cancer for 7 years. Educated, professional, and in control of her life, she was a long-range planner.

> Jeanie was the executive secretary for a leading business in the community. Initially seen and successfully treated for a posterior pharyngeal cancer, she returned for a scheduled follow-up. Her PET scan revealed cancer had recurred and was wrapped around the great vessels supplying her brain. Jeanie had received the maximum dose of radiation, and further surgery was not an option. She had a prognosis of less than 6 months.
>
> Two weeks after receiving the bad news, Jeanie returned to the office to collect her records and have one last evaluation. Impeccably dressed and with her usual calm, almost aloof demeanor, she informed the staff she was returning north to her hometown to accept hospice care. Jeanie expressed that she felt she would be more comfortable even though no family lived there any longer. The encounter ended with polite goodbyes and handshakes.

The clinical significance of Jeanie's diagnosis paled compared to her need to maintain her values and public persona. Her desire to be remembered as the competent professional she had been all of her life was important. Her history would be preserved.

While clinical success connotes a cure of the disease process, Relational Care recognizes that may not be the primary goal in every case. Care of the Body must be integrated with recognition and care of the Mind and Spirit for optimal results.

Questions for Reflection

1   Many Clinicians view treatment as a weapon in the warfare of disease. How do you envision your role in the fight? What is role of the Patient? What is the role of the Family?

2   Your long-term Patient is now terminal. How do you feel when you have to recommend hospice?

Reference

Siegel, B. (1998). *Peace, love, and healing.* Collins Publishers.

4

MIND

Objectives

1 Define the Mind
2 Describe the process of reframing
3 Understand the relationship of the Mind with the Body and Spirit

Introduction

Mind is the second element of Personhood. The thinking part of who we is is the activity of the brain. Specific areas of the brain control specific functions of the mind (Figure 4.1). However, not all functions of the mind can be explained by neurobiology. The mind is not a physical entity.

The hippocampus is part of the limbic system, critical in learning and memory. It consolidates information and associates memories with emotions. The anterior

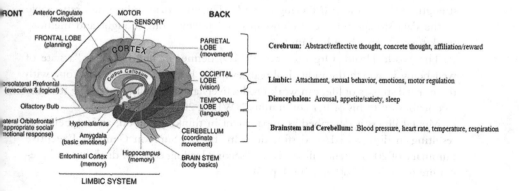

FIGURE 4.1   Schematic representation of brain function

DOI: 10.4324/9781003257219-6

cingulate controls normal emotions. Strong emotions are controlled by the amygdala, the center for emotional response to specific stimuli.

The orbitofrontal cortex and medial prefrontal cortex regulate human emotion and social behavior. In other words, large areas of brain are involved in the analysis of data *and* the emotional response to that process. The Mind is more complex than brain function alone.

Definition

Medical, mental health, and psychiatric professions have their own definitions of the Mind. Medically, altered mental status is an indication of physical injury or disease of the brain. The Mind is assessed by the Mini–Mental Status Exam (MMSE) and other cognitive assessments, while the brain is examined by CT, MRI, etc. Addressing the physical causes of mental illness is within the medical purview.

Mental health professions also use the MMSE as an evaluation tool. They focus on the ability to think, feel, perceive, and process. While aware of the impact of physical injury and disease, mental health professionals concentrate on psychological and emotional well-being. Practitioners appropriately use talk therapy with or without psychotropic medications.

Sigmund Freud (1923) includes preconscious, subconscious, and conscious thought as his psychiatric definition of the Mind. Presently, lack of insurance reimbursement has relegated psychiatry to pharmacotherapy.

Intelligence is the capacity and ability to think, reason, understand, learn, and create. There are different types of intelligence. Quantifying these are measured by testing for different factors.

Conscious and unconscious thought generate awareness and response to stimuli. The medical delineation between the two is well defined with specific terms including obtundent, stuporous, and lethargic. Even in a comatose state, there is brain activity.

The Mind receives input and associates it *with and into* pre-existing memories. Memory is the result of learning from an experience. Emotions reinforce and strengthen the memory (McGaugh, 2013). This information becomes retrievable in the data storage function. Conscious and unconscious thought and memory work together in a healthy Mind.

The World Health Organization (WHO) defines mental health as "a state of well-being in which the individual realizes his or her own abilities, can cope with the normal stresses of life, can work productively and fruitfully, and is able to make a contribution to his or her community" (WHO, 2018, p. 1).

Mental illness is described as impairment in thinking, mood, and/or behavior resulting in distress and/or dysfunction. In the US Surgeon General's Executive Summary of 2000, mental illness is the "second leading cause of disability and premature mortality" (Satcher, 2000, p. 5).

When the Mind is struggling, flat affect, slowed speech, and unkempt appearance might lead to a diagnosis of depression. The Beck Depression Inventory may support the diagnosis. However, many other factors may cause depressive symptoms. Substance use, legal or not, Family Dynamics, medications, burnout, etc., may lead to an incomplete or incorrect diagnosis. The classic clinical treatment for a mental health complaint is medication. However, research has shown that talk therapy, with or without medical therapy, is more efficacious (Hagen et al., 2010).

The choice of specialty within mental health professions may be confusing. Determining the etiology may require assessment and evaluation by a psychiatrist, who would manage the psychotropic medications. Clinical psychologists, Marriage and Family Therapists, Clinical Social Workers, Licensed Professional Counselors, Clinical Nurse Specialists, and Licensed Mental Health Counselors have training in a variety of subspecialties. Therapeutic options include Cognitive Behavioral, Dialectic Behavioral, Trauma, Substance Abuse, Addictions Therapies, and others.

Process

Each person visualizes an event differently. Within an experience, the Mind "reframes" events into a history that rationalizes and justifies perceptions and reactions. As time passes, memory of an event changes even more as the Mind transfers information into long-term memory.

Police reports and operational debriefs understand this tendency. Interrogations and debriefs occur as soon as possible after an event. Individuals give their version (usually separately and privately) to skilled interrogators. The compiled histories create a more accurate picture of what happened.

The conscious and unconscious Mind reasons and intuits. Logically, reason is conscious thought, used to understand and form judgment. Intuition is the experience of "knowing without knowing" that unconsciously uses cognitive and logical processes. Also known as a "sixth sense" or "trusting your gut," it is recognized as reliable. For example, many Clinicians close their eyes while palpating or auscultating to intensify concentration. This allows sense perception to be amplified by stored learning. Data, including knowledge, intellect, sense perception, and intuition, are synthesized.

Integration

The reality of "mind over matter" is not magic. It demonstrates the power that the Mind has in relationship with the Body and the Spirit. The Personal System recognizes the importance of Mind and Spirit collaborating with the Body for optimal health.

BOX 4.1 ABBY, MIKE, JOHN, AND JENNIFER

Just as memory is a function of the Mind, it contributes to sense of self. Behaviors and actions result within this context.

> While on a double date, Abby, John, Mike, and Jennifer heard a car crash right behind them. Abby, a nurse, and Mike, a police officer, ran to help. John, a combat veteran, ducked and looked for cover. Jennifer, a secretary, was startled and paralyzed.

Abby and Mike reacted as first responders. John reacted as a trained soldier under attack. Jennifer was confused and frozen in place by the suddenness of events. What we do and how we do it reflects our sense of self. The input was exactly the same for all four. Their responses reflected the Mindset of each individual.

Mindset is influenced by more than basic sensory input. Other organs and organ systems, namely, the adrenal, cardiac, respiratory, and gastrointestinal, influence the processing of data. This input can be negative or positive. Abbey, Mike, John, and Jennifer experienced "fight or flight." This physiological response reveals their Mindsets.

Studies trumpet the success and power of the Mind and Spirit's ability to effect "miracles" (World Federation for Mental Health, 2004). Little attention is paid to how Body, Mind, and Spirit *collaborate* to achieve these amazing results. The Body slows the heartbeat, reducing rate and pressure. The Mind focuses on breathing, reducing anxiety. The Spirit, sourcing inner healing and comfort, attains peace.

As powerful as the Body, Mind, Spirit interaction may be, dysfunction also has power.

Questions for Reflection

1   Psychiatry and psychotherapy are specialties that focus on diagnosis and treatment of the Mind. What factors would prompt you to request a psychiatric consult?

2   In addition to the Mini–Mental Status Exam (MMSE), how do you assess your Patients' mental health?

References

Freud, S. (1923). *The ego and the id.* Hogarth Press.

Gamon, D. (2016). *Your brain and what it does.* Allen D. Bragdon Publishers. Electronically retrieved from brainwaves.com.

Hagen, B., Wong-Wylie, G., & Pijl-Zieber, E. (2010). Tablets or talk? A critical review of the literature comparing antidepressants and counseling for treatment of depression. *Journal of Mental Health Counseling, 32*(2), 102–124. https://doil.org/10.17744/mehc.32.2.al84578m4137768k.

McGaugh, J. (2013). Making lasting memories: Remembering the significant. *Proceedings of the National Academy of the Sciences of the United States of America, 110*(Supplement 2), 10402–10407. https://doi.org/10.1073/pnas.13011209110.

Satcher, D. (2000). Mental health: A report of the surgeon general-executive summary. *Professional Psychology: Research and Practice, 31*(1), 5–13. https://doi.org/10.1037/0735-7028.31.1.5.

World Federation for Mental Health. (2004). *World mental health day. The relationship between physical and mental health: Co-occurring disorders.* Alexandria World Federation for Mental Health.

World Health Organization. (2018). *Mental health: Strengthening our response* (p. 1). World Health Organization Fact Sheet. Electronically retrieved from who.int/news-room/fact-sheets/detail/mental-health-strengthening-our-response.

5

SPIRIT

Objectives

1 Define Spirit
2 Describe suffering and differentiate it from pain
3 Understand what comprises a spiritual history

Introduction

Spirit is a necessary component of who and what we are. An amorphous element of personhood, it interprets, evaluates, rationalizes, and integrates experiences. Spirit is the source of passion, creativity, integrity, and hope. Not obviously housed in a particular organ, Spirit is more than an expression of the Mind and/or the heart (McCraty & Childre, 2004).

Spirituality is the "practice" of the Spirit that is unique to each individual. It may be seen as commonplace and comforting, intimidating and confusing, and/or disconcerting and unnecessary. Spirituality is more than a sense of self, or a sense of self in relation to others. It is awareness of relationship with the world.

As the Spirit matures, personal belief systems evolve. Individuals choose which practices and beliefs are integrated into their Spiritual formation. Depth and understanding of ones' place in the world evolves through experiences and learning. The many layers of spirituality are similar to Russian Matryoshka dolls – one doll inside of a larger doll, inside of even a larger doll. Each layer of growth and understanding generates a larger, more spiritually mature person.

Spirituality is not a trainable skill or easily defined. Educated in physiology and trained in the technology of medicine, Clinicians focus on cure and restoration of bodily health. The Body is tangible, easily accessed, and available. Testing and evaluation of it is relatively simple and straightforward. The Mind is more

DOI: 10.4324/9781003257219-7

complex. Testing and evaluation of the brain, where the Mind is housed, is difficult. Advanced imaging, computer modeling, and neuropsychiatric evaluations reveal new data on the functioning of the Mind. In contrast, there is no empiric testing and evaluation of Spirit.

Emotions are an integral part of the person and manifestation of Spirit. A product of the Mind, emotions derive from intellect and behavior. They influence multiple organ systems, including cardiovascular, pulmonary, adrenal, and gastrointestinal (McCraty & Childre, 2004).

Emotional response to loss is easily recognized. Compassion, empathy, forgiveness, anger, confusion, resentment, feeling of abandonment, isolation, fear, anxiety, hope, and love are experienced by Patient, Family, and Clinician. Emotions have no positive or negative value. They are the Spirit revealed.

Definition

The National Institute of Healthcare Research created a panel to define spirituality. Using experts in religion and spirituality, the panel defined it as "the feelings, thoughts, experiences, and behaviors that arise from a search for the sacred" (Young & Koopsen, 2005, p. 8). Spirituality has also been described as a connection to something or someone greater than oneself.

The analogy of a tapestry represents the formation of values. Values, the thread creating the tapestry, dictate the principles guiding behavior. They form personal morals and ethics. As our "moral compass," spiritual values influence decisions. Knowledge, present and historical, and the sense of what is right and wrong develop. Relationships, expectations, and connections clarify choices. The motivation for action is caring. Choices and actions result in consequential emotions. These are the expression of the Spirit.

Connections bridge past to future as they create the image of the tapestry. Each interweaves individuals, groups, generations (living and deceased), nature, art, religion, music, etc. Intuition, "trusting your gut," knowing without knowing, and having a "sixth sense" are manifestations of the tapestry of the Spirit.

Spirituality is a "multidimensional phenomenon" including concepts from theology, psychology, sociology, and medicine as demonstrated in Table 5.1. Spirituality influences the decisions we make and the behavior we exhibit. Another definition of spirituality is that which allows a person to experience transcendent meaning in life (Puchalski, 2006). This transcendence is the belief in the universe, a greater omniscient power (God), community with humanity, nature, music, and art.

Often mistaken for participation in religious practices, spirituality is a personally defined entity that informs how and why we live. "The spiritual nature of the person is broader than . . . organized religion" (Mahoney & Graci, 1999). Although the two are often used interchangeably, spirituality and religion are distinctly different. Someone may be religious without being spiritual or spiritual without being religious. Religion, as defined by Rousseau (2000), is a structured belief system

TABLE 5.1 Theories of Spirituality

Theological	Belief in God, expressed in religious beliefs and practices
Psychological	Expression of personal internal motives and desires
Sociological	Spiritual beliefs, practices, and rituals in personal relationships and in groups
Medical	Incorporating spiritual needs within medical plans

Source: Adapted from Young and Koopsen (2005)

addressing spiritual issues. Religion reflects the practice of spirituality through individual and community rituals (Klass, 1993).

Research has shown that a Patient's spirituality has significant impact on health. Puchalski (2006) reports that Patients with terminal illness benefit from spiritual growth and developing a sense of purpose. Confronting mortality is spiritually challenging for Patient, Family, and Clinician. Studies show that patients with developed, consistent spiritual practices have an improved response to stress and tend to live longer (Ellis & Campbell, 2004).

The correlation is unmistakable. Patients with spiritual well-being cope better with illness. They accept their illness, live well despite symptoms, and accept their impending death better than those who do not (Szaflarski et al., 2012).

A broken or "sick" Spirit may be the cause of intense pain that cannot be addressed medically. Although treatment of a "sick" Spirit is generally beyond the skills of most medical Clinicians, awareness of spiritual distress may improve Patient care and comfort. Collaboration with appropriately trained personnel (therapist, chaplain, etc.) will facilitate healing. Each person's Spirit determines their response to disease and compliance with treatment. Like the individual biochemical response to pharmaceuticals, the response of the Spirit to illness is unique.

BOX 5.1 CYNTHIA

Cynthia was an 82-year-old diabetic with End-Stage Renal Disease. She had been in and out of the hospital for months with recurrent infections and poor control of her comorbidities. As her body declined, her suffering during dialysis intensified. Despite the unit's best efforts, dialysis became a 12+ hour ordeal. Hypotension during each session would require halting dialysis, Trendelenberg positioning, and additional measures, to maintain a somewhat normal blood pressure.

Her most recent admission was for another urinary tract infection. However, her exam also revealed a new, ominous finding of dry gangrene of the left foot. Surgery was consulted, but the indicated amputation could not be safely done. As the gangrene slowly progressed up her leg, she told the dialysis unit she did not want to continue with treatment.

Her providers were duly notified and after formal consultation, Cynthia signed a DNR, including suspension of dialysis. As soon as her extensive family was informed of her decision, a vicious cycle began. The family descended, en masse, to Cynthia's hospital room and pressured her into revoking the DNR. Cynthia returned to dialysis, where family was not allowed. There, she wept and begged for treatment to stop. The staff obtained the EOL consultation and, once again, she signed the DNR. This cycle continued until her hospitalist requested an ethics consult for futility of care.

The next day, the hospitalist received an update from the chaplain who responded to the ethics consult request. The chaplain talked to Cynthia and her family, both separately and together. He was unable to obtain a DNR but was bringing in the family's minister later that day.

That meeting was long and difficult. But, without a Clinician in sight, a DNR was signed and supported by the family. Cynthia was allowed to transfer to hospice where she died comfortably a short time later.

Cynthia's pain was physical, mental, and spiritual. She wanted to stop the torture of dialysis, even though it would end her life. Her family suffered because they could not bear the thought of losing their mother, grandmother, sister, aunt. The medical team experienced the pain of futile treatment. Nurses cried with Cynthia as they prepared her for dialysis. The entire Healthcare Collaboration suffered.

The central factor in Cynthia's dying was not being addressed. Medicine could not help, but the chaplain was able to recognize the "therapy" needed for resolution. Inviting the Family's spiritual leader into the Healthcare Collaboration allowed him to advocate for Cynthia. Through him, her voice was heard and understood by her Family. The minister's spiritual support was necessary to make appropriate decisions regarding her Body.

Pain is different for each individual and not limited to nerve stimulation. The etiology of pain and suffering needs to be determined. If physical pain is the cause of discomfort, medications may be adjusted. Every Clinician is trained to diagnose and treat the causes of physical pain.

Patients experiencing generalized, indistinct pain may be suffering mental and/or spiritual distress. Depression, withdrawal, "giving up," or loss of hope builds — even when recovery is possible. If anxiety or fear is causing suffering, addressing the fear alleviates symptoms. Without human connections, discouragement develops.

Spirit cannot be discussed without acknowledging the meaning of suffering. Some patients may agonize over the "why?" or "why me?" Some find meaning and value in their suffering. Patients may view it as a redemptive act for previous wrongdoings, a trial of strength and resilience, or a testimony of their religious beliefs. In this "redemptive" suffering, the patient's tolerance for discomfort may be astonishingly high. Viktor Frankl's *Man's Search for Meaning* described concentration camp victims. Believing a purpose in their suffering increased their ability to endure inhumane treatment. This quality gave purpose to horror, making the "intolerable, tolerable." In refusing to accept their victimhood, Holocaust victims redefined their experience and gave value to their suffering (Frankl, 2006).

Kubler-Ross (1969) made the cogent point that medical technology has made suffering meaningless. The isolation of the hospitalized patient, especially in ICU, makes connection with family and friends difficult. It compounds spiritual suffering.

Additional areas of spiritual pain are generated in the Patients' journey through hope and forgiveness. Initially, the Patient hopes for a cure. Hope morphs into reaching a specific milestone or a pain-free death. Forgiving and the need to be forgiven alleviate spiritual pain and brings peace.

Without a relationship between Patient and Clinician, much less Family, in times of crisis, the Clinician is limited to medical data. Medical teams rely on protocols as opposed to conversations. Cynthia's medical condition changed the relationships within the Healthcare Collaboration. Once her suffering was identified and addressed, relationships were repaired. Cynthia's wishes were honored. Medicine was not able to cure Cynthia's Body; however, relationships were healed. The minister alleviated suffering for her and the entire Healthcare Collaboration.

Process

"Spirituality is not a thing or a state of being, but is a process of interaction" (Klass, 1993, p. 51). The use of "process" does not refer to stages or phases. The Body and the Mind experience while the Spirit interprets and feels the impact.

Spiritual growth is necessary for both maturity and progression toward a peaceful acceptance of mortality. Crisis creates opportunity for spiritual growth and maturation. Puchalski (2006) describes this reflection as LIFE.

"L" stands for *Life Review* where choices, accomplishments, offences, and hurts are reviewed. The review is reframed in the Patient's memory, granting meaning and peace. "I" refers to *Identity* – as the Patient defines who they are and their role in life. "F" is *Forgiveness and Reconciliation*. Forgiveness, being at peace with oneself, with others, and with "God," has been known to impact health. "E" represents *Eternity*, the person's beliefs regarding what happens after death. Even for those who do not express a belief in afterlife, there is the strong need to be remembered and cared for after they are gone.

Clinicians need to be cognizant of spiritual issues. Acknowledging and recognizing spiritual distress facilitates referral to the appropriate spiritual or mental health counselor. Table 5.2 lists many common spiritual issues faced by Patients, Families, *and* Clinicians.

TABLE 5.2 Some Spiritual Issues Faced by Patients

Spiritual Issues
Lack of meaning and purpose
Hopelessness
Despair
Not being remembered
Guilt/shame
Anger at God/others
Abandonment by God/others
Feeling out of control
Spiritual pain/suffering
Mistrust
Lack of forgiveness/reconciliation

Source: Adapted from Puchalski and Ferrell (2010)

Spirituality within the practice of medicine is the recognition and appreciation of our own spirituality as well as the spirituality of others. This ability, this
connection, may be lacking in health care. Impersonal practice of medicine leaves
Patients dissatisfied with care. "Professional" behavior is taught as a form of protective distancing in medicine. Consequentially, the Healthcare Collaboration can
experience distress.

The Clinician who has confronted his or her own mortality is open to fuller
connection and communication with their Patients. This openness can lead to
healing even in the face of death.

BOX 5.2 ED

Clinicians need to be aware that spirituality affects decisions in care, living,
and dying. Often the professional who does not pay attention to the "whole"
Patient has "an incomplete understanding of illness" (Siegel, 1998).

*At 98 years of age, Ed had Parkinson's Disease, bladder cancer, and pros-
tate cancer. A WWII veteran, his spine was partially fused with osteoarthri-
tis. His increasing pain made walking difficult. His family pressured him
to walk, eat properly, and take physical therapy to improve his strength.
In frustration, he fired the physical therapist. When confronted with his
"rude" behavior, he explained (again) that he was done. He was tired
and ready to die.*

*Finally listening, the family acquiesced to hospice care. Ed was pleased.
He reminded his loved ones that he had lived a full life and was ready*

> *to die. Once in hospice, Ed used his wheelchair exclusively. His diet was*
> *no longer restricted and he began to improve. He gained weight, became*
> *more alert, and complained less. Hospice remarked that he was showing*
> *signs of doing so well, they were considering "firing" him.*
>
> Ed spent his life in control of himself. During his illness, his family co-opted
> his Spirit by insisting on dictating his daily activities regarding nutrition and
> physical therapy. His family wanted him to be physically well. Their desire to
> cure his Body was understandable, yet unattainable. He declined, not because
> of his physical condition alone but because of his sick Spirit. Once he reas-
> serted control over his Body and Mind, his Spirit renewed.
>
> Ed was not cured, but his Mind and his Spirit were healed. He expressed
> appreciation for his life. His Family accepted the natural decline of his Body. He
> became comfortable in Body, Mind, and Spirit. He flourished for the remain-
> ing 6 months of his life.

Patients have expressed a desire to connect spiritually with their Clinician. As
Clinicians focus on the scientific method and pathophysiology of the disease process, the Patient as a person becomes secondary. The dissociation between the
person and the disease process widens as another protective mechanism.

The belief in something greater than ourselves increases our awareness and
accountability. The spiritually mature recognize death as part of the natural cycle
of life. That is not to say that the spiritual seek death, but they find peace with it.
Belief in an afterlife is not necessary.

Integration

Knowing that we are Body, Mind, *and* Spirit enables us to appreciate how value
systems are generated. Life is experienced through the Body. Intellectual yearning involves the Mind. Processed by the Mind, the Spirit interprets, judges, and
gives value and meaning. The Spirit can be consciously expanded and disciplined,
through study and meditation, or developed through life experience. By respecting
another's values, Spirit is honored.

Spiritual growth is not dependent on a specific discipline or practice. Being open
to experiences and thoughtful contemplation expands the meaning of life. Values
are enriched and formed with spiritual maturity. Clarity in decision-making grows
when we pay attention to the spiritual. "All respondents [Patients] viewed spirituality as a healing resource, considering spiritual and physical health closely connected"
(Ellis & Campbell, 2004). It takes awareness, openness, and self-confidence to follow one's instincts and heart. It takes courage to step outside the boundaries of
standardized protocol. "Being," not "doing," manifests Clinician's Spirit.

Patient and Family suffering requires quiet observation by the Clinician. Listening to what and how Patients describe their feelings reveals physiological and nonphysiological suffering. When Patients complain of symptoms grossly exaggerated compared to their physical examination findings, a "red flag" is waving. Other Patients may assert they are "fine" when they obviously are not. It takes presence and unusual patience to discern the cause of suffering.

Listening to the silences is helpful. Listening, being present, is difficult in the linear thinking, time pressured, medical mindset. Clinicians must appreciate how disease impacts Personhood. Acknowledging "spiritual interests" is the first step in learning what is needed to incorporate care of the Spirit into the Healthcare Collaboration (Patient, Family, and Clinician). Treating a physical complaint and moving on ignores the opportunity to heal holistically.

While it may be defined or perceived in different ways, spirituality is common in all persons. The connections among humans exist on many levels and from many different perspectives. Dr. Naomi Remen (1999) summarized her philosophy on life/spirituality in this manner:

> *Helping, fixing, and serving represent three different ways of seeing life. When you help, you see life as weak. When you fix, you see life as broken. When you serve, you see life as whole. Fixing and helping may be the work of the ego. Service is work of the soul.*

Spiritual connection and service transcend boundaries – economic, mental, physical, and social. The very fabric of our Personhood is woven with these interrelationships. It is a tapestry of our lives that transcends death.

Questions for Reflection

1   "Someone may be religious without being spiritual or spiritual without being religious." How does that statement resonate with you?
2   Think of a time when you encountered a "sick" Spirit. How were you changed by this experience?

References

Ellis, M., & Campbell, J. (2004). Patients' views about discussing spiritual issues with primary care physicians. *Southern Medical Journal, 97*(12), 1158–1164.

Frankl, V. (2006). *Man's search for meaning.* Beacon Press.

Klass, D. (1993). Spirituality, Protestantism, and death. In K. Doka & J. Morgan (Eds.), *Death and spirituality* (p. 51). J. Baywood Publishing.

Kubler-Ross, E. (1969). *On death and dying.* MacMillan Publishing.

Mahoney, M., & Graci, G. (1999). The meanings and correlates of spirituality: Suggestions from an exploratory survey of experts. *Death Studies.* Taylor and Francis, *23*, 521–528.

McCraty, R., & Childre, D. (2004). The grateful heart. In R. Emmons & M. McCollough (Eds.), *The psychology of gratitude* (pp. 230–254). Oxford University Press.

Puchalski, C. (2006). *A time for listening and caring.* Oxford University Press.

Puchalski, C., & Ferrell, B. (2010). *Making health care whole.* Templeton Press.

Remen, R. (1999). Helping, fixing or serving? *Shambhala Sun.* Electronically retrieved October 3, 2021, from www.mentalhealthsf.org

Rousseau, P. (2000). Spirituality and the dying patient. *Journal of Clinical Oncology, 18*(9), 2000–2002.

Siegel, B. (1998). *Peace, love, and healing* (p. 119). Collins, Publishers.

Szaflarski, M., Kundel, I., Cotton, S., Leonard, A., Tsevat, J., & Ritchey, P. (2012). Multi-dimensional assessment of spirituality/religion in patients with HIV: Conceptual framework and empirical refinement. *Journal of Religion and Health, 51,* 1239–1260.

Young, C., & Koopsen, C. (2005). *Spirituality, health, and healing.* SLACK Incorporated.

6

RELATIONAL SYSTEM

Objectives

1 Define Patient, Family, and Clinician
2 Review the Personal System and the Relational System

Introduction

The Relational System is formed by the relationship of the Patient, Family, and Clinician. The functioning and responsibility of members of this system is the Healthcare Collaboration. The Relational System is larger than the Personal System, with indistinct and amorphous borders. While the Mind and Spirit are not well defined, Patient, Family, and Clinician are easier to understand.

Definition

Of the three elements in the Relational System, the Patient is the most easily defined. The center of attention and, hopefully, the director of their personal story, the Patient is the reason the Relational System exists. The ability of the Patient to express their wishes and "direct their movie" can vary with the health and well-being of their Personhood.

Families provide an excellent example of how systems work. One person's Family may be a huge extended tribe including cousins, uncles, and in-laws. Conversely, another Family may be a significant other or a lifelong close friend. No matter what the Patient's definition of their Family is, the unit must be respected as such.

DOI: 10.4324/9781003257219-8

BOX 6.1 ERNEST

Ernest was the elderly "ambassador of the neighborhood." His Yorkie, Max, was Ernest's bodyguard, always with him. They were often seen touring the neighborhood by bicycle, with Max perched in a special basket. As they both aged, the tours were completed in a convertible sports car, with Max riding in style on the folded top. Max was very protective of Ernest, barking and threatening anyone who came near "his human." The neighbors knew Max would snap if he did not approve.

Angela, Ernest's wife, and Max had a difficult relationship. Despite his small size, Max considered himself the alpha male, dominant over Angela. He would tolerate her occasional pets. But he had been known to snap at her, especially if she tried to pick him up. They maintained an uneasy peace, with their mutual love of Ernest their only common ground.

Ernest suffered a stroke. Angela was told he was comatose and not going to recover. In the days following, Angela noticed Max moping, with poor appetite and little energy. She tried to get him out on walks, but neither seemed to be enjoying the activity. Both were grieving.

At Ernest's bedside a few days later, Angela mentioned Max's failure to thrive to the nurse, Charlotte. Knowing Ernest was scheduled for discharge to hospice soon, Charlotte "suggested" that Max could be smuggled into the hospital for a final visit with his "Dad." With a few suggestions on how to keep the expedition deniable to the staff, Angela decided to do it.

When she arrived home early that evening, she started talking to Max. Using her family name for Ernest, "Daddy," Angela talked to Max as she tried to coax him into eating something. Max perked his ears at the word, "Daddy," but resumed moping when Ernest did not appear. With trepidation, Angela approached the dog, stating repetitively, "Let's go see Daddy." She was stunned when Max allowed her to pick him up and take him to the car.

Once at the hospital, Angela admonished Max. She told him he could not bark or fight to get out of the large purse she used to carry him. She smuggled Max into Ernest's room without incident. Placed on the bed, Max immediately sniffed his way up to Ernest's chest and laid down under his chin. Occasionally lifting his head to sniff, Max was content and amazingly quiet. When it was time to leave, Max was quiet and noncombative. Subsequently, Max began eating and bonding with Angela.

Charlotte and Angela recognized Max as a beloved family member. All were grieving their losses. Angela was transitioning to living without Ernest, while Max was transitioning to a new life without "Daddy."

The definition of a Clinician is a healthcare provider at any level, from patient care technician to attending physician. Many Patients and Families see one provider as "their doctor" and are confused and surprised by a multidisciplinary team. In an already confusing and stressful environment, keeping track of the lead physician, the consulting team, the advanced providers, nursing, various therapists, etc. is virtually impossible.

In the Family's eyes, the Clinician can be viewed as the imminent authority figure, a knowledgeable ally, or, at best, a partner in the care of their loved one. As one Family member observed to a Clinician, "There are so many of you taking care of Dad, I need a playbook!"

Process

The goal of the Relational System (Patient, Family, Clinician), through the function of the Healthcare Collaboration, is to reach consensus. How effective and successful this System operates depends on contributing variables. It is easy to identify members of each element. Recognizing the *effect* of each on the other is a greater challenge. This requires understanding and respecting values and priorities. Clear communication is critical to promoting consensus.

Integration

The Healthcare Collaboration does not exist without all three elements. Obviously, the Patient is the "sick one." The composition of the Family, defined by the Patient, are those in relationship with him or her. The value and the importance of the relationship may be interpreted differently by each member. The Clinician is the designated expert and authority in matters of disease and/or injury. The expectation that Clinicians have the "power" to fix everything is unrealistic.

Relational Care recognizes the process of change within the Personal and Relational Systems together. The dynamic, nonlinear interactions occur simultaneously, resulting in change itself.

Returning to the analog watch (Figure 2.1) illustrates how all elements interact. The Relational System is composed of multiple gears operating *in synch*. Function or dysfunction in one impacts all of the others. Each Body, Mind, Spirit (Personal System) is necessarily a member of the Patient, Family, and Clinician (Relational System).

BOX 6.2   STEPHEN

The Healthcare Collaboration is formed by personhoods, working together. This process is complex and fluid.

During Stephen's coronary artery bypass grafting, the damage was more extensive than expected. His postoperative course was rocky, and the staff could not wean him off the ventilator and pressors. His prognosis was grim.

The resident, Robert, tried to prepare Francine, Stephen's wife, for the worst. As they discussed his prognosis, she began to cry. Francine left the foot of the bedside and went to stroke Stephen's head. She leaned over, kissed his cheek, and whispered into his ear. Robert watched in astonishment at the foot of the bed, as Stephen's blood pressure and pulse began to normalize. As the days progressed, he was weaned off the ventilator and medications.

Once on the floor and readying for discharge, Robert brought up the extraordinary moment to the couple. Stephen had no memory of the incident. Robert asked Francine what she said before the dramatic recovery. Blushing and refusing to meet his eyes, she replied, "I love you, you son of a bitch. If you die on me, I'm going to KILL you!"

Relationships are powerful medicine.

The strength of the Relational System depends upon the awareness and appreciation of the values of each member. Relational Care makes sense of the relationships between both the Personal System and Relational System to the benefit of all.

Questions for Reflection

1   List the families you belong to.
2   Draw a large circle and place a small circle labeled "you" in the center. Position the names of family, friends, co-workers, etc. within the circle according to their value to you.

PART III
Barriers and Baggage

7

DYING AND DEATH

Objectives

1 Define death
2 Describe the characteristics of transition
3 Understand the stages and tasks of dying
4 Describe "a good death"

Introduction

Dying is difficult for everyone. Whether sudden and unexpected, or at the end of a prolonged illness, it is unbalancing, confusing, and disorienting. A terminal diagnosis forces change in the structure of the Healthcare Collaboration. This restructuring is experienced physically, mentally, spiritually, emotionally, socially, and financially. The first of many changes takes place as roles shift.

In surveys of Patients and Clinicians alike, fear of dying alone predominates (Gavrin, 2007). The timing of a Patient's last breath and heartbeat is influenced by numerous factors – many outside the parameters of medical science. For example, dying Patients may wait for certain family members to arrive. Other deaths may occur within minutes of the Family leaving the bedside.

Dying is anathema to Clinicians. They do not concede, viewing death as defeat. There is little education on communicating with dying Patients and their Families. There is even less research on dying and death. Taking care of the caregiver strategies is virtually nonexistent.

Definitions of Death

The definition of death has changed. The classic definition is cessation of spontaneous cardiopulmonary activity. It remains the general public's understanding

DOI: 10.4324/9781003257219-10

of death. Science and technology necessitated changes. Organ transplantation created the need for a new definition as medical teams sustain cardiopulmonary activity until surgery. Ethically, most organs may not be harvested from a "living" human being. Revised definitions of death were developed and legally adopted as improved monitoring and support of vital functions evolved.

Brain death, medically known as "total brain failure" (TBF), is defined as irreversible cessation of *whole* brain function (National Conference of Commissioners on Uniform State Laws, 1980). TBF allows the harvest of organs from bodies while maintaining and sustaining cardiopulmonary function.

Higher brain death, also known as neocortical death, is yet another medical definition. Loss of brain responsible for consciousness, memory, personality, and perception, with preservation of hindbrain function, constitutes neocortical death (Zaner, 1988). In higher brain death, body function regulation and primitive reflexes are typically preserved, and interaction with the environment is nonexistent. This is often seen in Patients who sustain hypoxic brain injury. A nationwide inpatient study of those who survived CPR and hypoxic brain injury reported 77.9% died in the hospital and 14% were discharged to a long-term care facility (Allareddy et al., 2015).

BOX 7.1 JAHI

Multiple definitions, combined with technology, create the basis for many End-of-Life conflicts.

Jahi McMath was a 13-year-old girl with pediatric obstructive sleep apnea. She underwent an adenotonsillectomy, uvulectomy, and turbinectomy on December 9, 2013. Postoperatively, she was alert and oriented in the pediatric ICU. There, she hemorrhaged acutely and coded. Despite efforts to control the hemorrhage and her airway, she suffered an anoxic event.

Her parents were unable to accept the diagnosis of brain death. Numerous consults, including a pediatric neurologist, determined that she had full, unrecoverable, loss of brain function. Although she had spontaneous cardiac activity, she had no control of respirations or temperature regulation. Her upper level functioning was nonexistent. On December 12, 2013, a formal death certificate was issued.

Her parents fought the diagnosis in the hospital, the press, and the courts. Although the hospital's stance on Jahi's condition never changed, the administration agreed to keep her on the ventilator until alternative care arrangements were made. Jahi was transferred to an undisclosed, private facility on January 5, 2014. There she received a tracheostomy and gastric feeding tube. She remained in her comatose state until her death on June 22, 2018.

Unable to find shared values regarding Jahi's death, the Healthcare Collaboration was nonfunctioning. Her parents believed their daughter was still "alive" while Clinicians declared her "dead."

Understanding the definitions of death is one of the first steps in contributing to a "good death." In today's society, death is taboo. The word death is avoided like a communicable disease. Language includes convenient euphemisms like "passing on," the "big sleep," or "didn't make it." Culturally, it evokes the power of prediction because the "D word" was spoken aloud. Necessary conversations are avoided (Davenport & Schopp, 2011), despite the need for Advance Directives and wills.

Witnessing death no longer takes place in daily life. Historically, as part of agrarian societies with high mortality rates, death was common. Dying in hospitals rather than dying at home, Patients are isolated in ICU without family members at bedside. Even the family pet is euthanized at the vet's office with the body discreetly disposed of – "out of sight, out of mind."

Clinicians are isolated from their dying Patient as well. Most hospitalized Patients are under a cadre of specialists' care. At End of Life (EOL), palliative care or hospice services are used, further excluding Clinicians from the process. Clinicians rarely experience a death outside of a failed Advanced Cardiac Life Support protocol. Death is seen as failure in the clinical setting. However, when death hits too close to home, everyone is blindsided.

Many people are aware of the terms "full code," "no code," and "Do Not Resuscitate (DNR)." There are multiple levels of "codes." Allow Natural Death (AND) is a relatively new term that is increasing in usage. POLST, originally known as Physician Orders for Life-Sustaining Treatment, is an order set for EOL care. It is based on the Patient's Advance Directives (AD). Code levels, POLST, and ADs are necessary because of the number of providers involved in Patient care and the need for clear communication.

Historically, death occurred within 24–48 hours after significant injury or illness. With today's technology, "the end of life can now last several years" (Puchalski, 2006). Active dying is clinically called transition.

Transition

The physiological process of the Body shutting down is termed transition. The pace of dying is variable and hard to predict. Disease severity is one influence in the speed of progression, which can be a rapid crash or slow decline.

The pre-active phase of transition is a gradual Patient withdrawal from most social interactions. No longer seeking visitors, Patients prefer to be quietly alone with a close loved one. Their appetite decreases or they stop eating. As they progress, they will refuse fluids and medication.

There are two forms of active transition – the quiet and the agitated. The quiet form is marked by a lethargic slide into a coma leading to death. Agitated transition is marked by restlessness, hallucinations, seizures, and delirium before lapsing into a coma and death. Both include multiple physical findings summarized in Table 7.1.

TABLE 7.1 Constellation of Symptoms Seen in Dying Patients

Time Before Demise	Sign or Symptom	Notes
Months to Weeks	Withdrawal from social interaction	Wanting only certain people to visit, depression
	Loss of Activities of Daily Living	Gradual loss of ability to self-care
	Decreased interest in food/ hydration	
	Cognitive changes – somnolence, delirium	Delirium with altered vital signs may indicate a treatable issue
	Nausea, vomiting, dry mouth, dysphagia, abdominal discomfort	Rule out medication causes
	Dyspnea, fatigue	Variable, rule out medications and treatable causes
Weeks to Days	Bedbound	
	Further decline in mental status, anxiety/depression	Slowed mentation
	Longer periods of time asleep	
	Reduced PO intake	May have difficulty with PO medication, even in liquid form
	Transient clinical improvement	Family will report a "good day" or rally
	Kennedy Terminal Ulcers	Rapid, irreversible skin breakdown as blood shunts to core
Days to Hours	Change in vital signs and mentation	Not associated with pre-existing conditions
	Oliguria or anuria	May not be present with pre-existing conditions
	Coma	Coma mixed with delirium, may be agitated

(Continued)

TABLE 7.1 (Continued)

Time Before Demise	Sign or Symptom	Notes
	Audible oral secretions, "death rattle"	Suctioning increases risk of aspiration
Hours to Minutes (Active transition)	Mottling and cooling of extremities	Livedo reticularis
	Alterations in vital signs	Hypotension and tachycardia as cardiac output slows
	Ileus, urinary retention	Fecal and/or urinary incontinence may occur
Minutes	Abnormal, terminal breathing pattern	Low tidal volume with agonal pattern and/or jaw thrusting
	Bradycardia and irregular rhythm	Pulse weakens, becomes more central, slow, and erratic

Source: Adapted from Haig (2009), Hui et al. (2015), and Weissman (2021)

Active transition is hallmarked by vague and chaotic signs and symptoms. There are no lab findings or diagnostic studies that prognosticate imminent demise. The lungs begin to fail leading to mottled, cool skin. Slowed respirations result in apneic episodes. The heart fails, causing pulmonary and hepatic congestion. The patient can hear but may not respond. There is decreased sensation. Response to touch diminishes.

The patient may retain or become incontinent of both feces and urine. Both conditions can cause discomfort and distress. Urinary output decreases and may become dark or contain blood. The pulse rate will remain strong while death is hours away. Once it becomes weak and irregular, death is imminent.

Kennedy Terminal Ulcers occur in the days preceding death. They are a result of blood shunting away from the periphery to the core of the Body. Often confused by Family with decubiti and poor care, these ulcers can be dressed but cannot be successfully treated. The tissue is irreversibly dying.

Sometimes in the dying process, the need for pain relief surpasses normal dosing. A lethal narcotic dose may barely touch the Patient's pain. The Rule of Double Effect allows for comfort care to take precedence over strict adherence to narcotic dosing. As long as the intent is to alleviate suffering, the action is ethical, even if it hastens demise. It is not euthanasia.

BOX 7.2 PHYLLIS

Without Advance Directives, emergency personnel and Family are placed in difficult positions when confronted with a family member/Patient in transition.

Phyllis arrived by ambulance, having passed out at a funeral. Her terminal state was obvious with her respiratory distress, grossly distended

> *abdomen, and cachectic limbs. Only after she was intubated, did the Cli-nicians discover she had stage IV ovarian cancer. Her only child, Amelia, aged 21, was brought in to make decisions regarding Phyllis' care.*
>
> *Amelia's aunt Lee and uncle Jim accompanied her to talk to the oncolo-gist. In the meeting, Amelia was anxious and tentative. Lee asked ques-tions on her behalf, hoping to confirm her sister's obvious terminal status. The oncologist retreated into medicalese in all of his responses. Finally, Lee asked directly, "Is the ventilator maintaining Phyllis' life?" Once the doctor clearly stated that Phyllis was terminal, Amelia was able to decide. The agreement was made to withdraw life support that night.*
>
> *Per Amelia's request, Family gathered at bedside while Phyllis was extu-bated. Prayers, songs, and stories were shared. The internist and oncolo-gist waited outside the room until the last heartbeat was registered, about 45 minutes later.*

Clinicians and Family were missing direction from Phyllis. Without Advance Directives, the Emergency Department was forced to code her. Amelia was caught in a whirlwind of grief and confusion. She was unable to make a decision.

Uncomfortable with the entire conversation, the oncologist retreated to medical jargon. Facilitated by Lee, clear, simple communication allowed the Healthcare Collaboration to reach consensus regarding Phyllis' care.

Stages and Tasks

Dying is hard work. Understanding the dying process gives insight into the perspec-tive of the dying Personhood. Dr. Elizabeth Kubler-Ross, in her pioneering book *On Death and Dying*, introduced her "stages" of dying (1969). Similar to the stages of grief, they include Denial, Anger, Bargaining, Depression, and Acceptance. These stages or behaviors are not experienced in any specific order and/or timeframe.

Denial may be demonstrated by isolation after the shock of "bad news." Differ-ent expressions of anger (at God, those who are well, medicine, etc.) are common and may occur at any time. Bargaining is a spiritual component. As an appeal to a higher power, it is an "if . . . then" conversation for change. Depression results from mourning present and future losses. Acceptance is resignation to the inevitability of the demise, usually marked by withdrawal and "giving up the fight" in peaceful resignation. Not all "stages" are experienced by every dying person.

Often described as "tasks of dying," "choices of dying" may be a more accurate descriptor. Care of the Body includes choosing treatments and site of care (home or institution). Caring of the Mind includes choosing to resolve unfinished business and saying goodbyes. Care of the Spirit includes choosing to make peace by giving and accepting forgiveness of self and others. These "tasks" are unique and personal (Worden, 2002).

Dollars and Sense

Technology impacts the finances of medicine, aging, and dying. Personal financial resources impact treatment compliance. Dying Patients sustain increased "expenditure and economic burden" with minimal change in overall outcome (Eid et al., 2017, pp. 13–20). Studies show that as the elder population explodes, more of the healthcare dollar is spent on chronically ill, elder Patients. A study by Knickman and Snell (2002) revealed that approximately $120 *billion*/year is spent in elder care. This figure is an underestimate, because the study did not include "informal" care delivered by Family and friends.

The financial impact of the COVID-19 pandemic will be studied for years to come. The personal cost, both from lost wages to hospitalization for care, have been financially devastating for many families. An analysis by Kaiser found that out-of-pocket costs for COVID medical care could exceed $1300 for patients with employer-based insurance (Wapner, 2020). Studies agree that the prolonged pandemic has contributed to financial volatility and wild fluctuations in markets (Albulescu, 2021). In a study comparing worldwide and US financial volatility, researchers concluded that worldwide fatalities contributed greatly to volatility.

Clinicians are taught the "gold standard," evidence-based medical treatment for disease. Many are unaware of the cost to the Patient, much less Family. Depending on insurance coverage and co-pay, costs may be minimal or exorbitant.

BOX 7.3 MELISSA

Many times, compliance is directly related to cost.

Melissa had been hospitalized for more than a week. At 72 years of age, her poorly controlled diabetes wreaked havoc on her Body. Despite optimization of care, the damage was extensive and permanent. She was wheelchair bound, had a permanent urinary catheter, and required nursing home placement.

In discussions with her Clinicians, Melissa expressed understanding and agreement with the treatment plan and need for placement. However, when discharge became imminent, another complication or complaint would arise. It gradually occurred to the treatment team that these "complications" were manufactured by Melissa.

Her social worker discovered that Melissa's invalid, elderly father, her daughter, and two young grandchildren depended on her disability status for both income and housing. If Melissa went into the nursing home, housing would be lost and her income would go to the nursing home. Upon learning this, the social worker arranged for expedited social services, including income and housing, for Melissa's family. Subsequently, she was transferred to the nursing home without further "complications."

> Melissa's Personal System expressed her fears through physical complaints. Her distress was due to her belief that she was "abandoning" her Family. Once her Family was provided for, Melissa's new complaints disappeared.

The elder population puts the greatest strain on the medical system. The overall disability of the average elder is improved compared to previous decades. However, chronic disease with increased longevity skyrockets healthcare costs.

"Most healthcare dollars are spent near the end of a person's life" (Chop, 2015, p. 13). A study of Emergency Department (ED) visits illustrates the "silver tsunami." As expected, elders hospitalized from the ED experienced significant rise in disabilities. Additionally, an ED visit without subsequent hospitalization resulted in a significant decline in overall health. Clinical decline in the following 6 months, without hospitalization, indicated a new vulnerability to the elder population with increased risk (Nagurney et al., 2017).

Over 75% of Americans now die in some form of institution, usually a hospital. However, most wish to die at home (Muramatsu et al., 2008). Over 80% of the average healthcare dollar is spent on the last 6 months of a Patient's life. The costs are exponentially higher with ICU admission. Many dying Patients are shuffled from one care facility to another as the dying process creeps along, when they prefer to be home. Despite demonstrated cost savings, insurances have been slow to cover palliative or hospice care (Meghani & Hinds, 2015). Aetna was the first company to recognize the cost-effectiveness of EOL care (Shesgreen, 2010). England's "tuck-in" service is covered by insurance and decreases overall cost because care is given by minimally trained nurses' aides. EOL discussions prevent suffering and save dollars.

Despite this recognized benefit, Clinicians are still slow in ordering palliative and hospice care. An international study in 2020 revealed that out of 23 countries, the average length of stay in a US palliative service before death was 19 days. In all other countries with palliative services, the length of stay averaged 29 days. This trend continues, despite evidence that quality of life *and* longevity is improved with palliative services (Jordan et al., 2020).

The "Good Death"

A "good death" appears to be an oxymoron. Albeit reluctantly, dying presents both Patient and Family with enormous growth opportunity. Priorities reorder. Relationships re-connect, repair, and re-establish. Authentic communication facilitates forgiveness of self and others. A good death offers summation and a finale to life — with growth, healing, and peace.

Most of us have intimate knowledge of a difficult death. This occurs with estrangement, incomplete grief work, and buried, unresolved guilt. Caregiving through the dying process, although overwhelming in scope, creates satisfying memories with loved ones. A good death develops with unique synergy involving multiple communities- Family, medical, religious/spiritual, neighborhood, social, and professional services. Throughout the process, interdependence and communication must remain open, clear, and available to all. The language of death must be clear. A "good death" is never as seamless as described.

A "good death" requires work and self-awareness. How one dies is influenced by two factors – how one lives and how one communicates. Choices, relationships, and values influence how death is viewed. A final battle fighting to the end, a doorway to the next life, or the end of one's existence and importance in the world have unique meaning. Dying and death reflect how we have lived and what we believe. Relational Care supports every member of the Healthcare Collaboration throughout the journey.

Questions for Reflection

1   There are three definitions of death in use today. What is yours?
2   What does a "good death" mean to you?

References

Albulescu, C. T. (2021). COVID-19 and the United States. *Financial Research Letters, 38*, 101699. https://doi.org/10.1016/j.frl.2020.101699

Allareddy, V., Rampa, S., Nalliah, R., Martinez-Schlurmann, N., Lidsky, K., Allareddy, V., & Rotta, A. (2015). Prevalence and predictors of gastrostomy tube placement in anoxic/hypoxic ischemic encephalopathic survivors of in-hospital cardiopulmonary resuscitation in the United States. *PLoS ONE.* https://doi.org/10.1371/journal.pone.0132612

Chop, W. (2015). Demographic trends of an aging society. In R. Robnett & W. Chop (Eds.), *Gerontology for the health care professional* (p. 13). Jones and Barlett Learning.

Davenport, L., & Schopp, G. (2011). Breaking bad news: Communication skills for difficult conversations. *Journal of American Academy of Physician Assistants, 24*(2), 46–50. https://doi.org/10.1097/01720610-201102000-00008

Eid, S., Abougergi, M., Albaeni, A., & Chandra-Strobos, N. (2017). Survival, expenditure, and disposition in patients following out of hospital cardiac arrest: 1995–2013. *Resuscitation, 113*, 13–20. https://doi.org/10/1016/j.resuscitation.2016.12.027

Gavrin, J. (2007). Ethical considerations at the end of life in the intensive care unit. *Critical Care Medicine, 35*(Supplement 2), S85–S94. https://doi.org/101097/01.CCM.0000252909.52316.27

Haig, S. (2009). Diagnosing dying: Symptoms and signs of end-stage disease. *End of Life Care, 3*(4), 8–12.

Hui, D., Dev, R., & Bruera (2015). The last days of life: Symptom burden and impact on nutrition and hydration in cancer patients. *Current Opinion Support Palliative Care, 9*(4), 346–354. https//doi.org/10.1097/SPC.0000000000000171

Jordan, R., Allsop, M., ElMokhallati, Y., Jackson, C., Edwards, H., Chapman, E. Duliens, L., & Bennett, M. (2020). Duration of palliative care before death in international routine practice: A systematic review and meta-analysis. *BMC Medicine, 18*, 368. https://doi.org/10.1186/s12916-020-01829-x

Knickman, J., & Snell, E. (2002). The 2030 problem: Caring for aging baby boomers. *Health Services Research, 17*(4), 849–884. https://doi.org/101034.j.1600-05602002.56.x

Kubler-Ross, E. (1969). *On dying and death*. Scribner.

Meghani, S., & Hinds, P. (2015). Policy brief: The institute of medicine report dying in America: Improving quality and honoring individual preferences near end of life. *Nursing Outlook, 63*(1), 51–59 https://doi.org/10/1016/j.outlook.2014.11.007

Muramatsu, N., Hoyem, R., Hongjun, Y., & Campbell, R. (2008). Place of death among older Americans. *Medical Care, 46*(8), 829–838. https://doi.org/10/1097/MLR.0b013e3181791a79

Nagurney, J., Fleischman, W., Han, L., Leo-Summers, L., Allore, H., & Gill, T. (2017). Risk factors for disability after emergency department discharge in older adults. *Academic Emergency Medicine, 27*(2), 1270–1278. https://doi.org/10/1111/acem.14088. PMID:32673434

National Conference of Commissioners on Uniform State Laws. (1980). *Uniform determination of death act*. uniformlaws.org/HigherLogic/System/DownloadDocumentFile. ashx?DocumentFilekey= 341343fa-1efe-706c-043a-9290fdcfd909

Puchalski, C. (2006). *A time for listening and caring*. Oxford University Press.

Shesgreen, D. (2010, October 7). Aetna led the way on "concurrent care". *The Connecticut Mirror*.

Wapner, J. (2020). COVID -19: Medical expenses leave many Americans deep in debt. *British Medical Journal, 370*. https://doi.org/10.1136/bmj.m3097 https://doi.org/10.1136/bmj.m3097

Weissman, D. (2021). *Fast facts and concepts #3 Syndrome of imminent death*. Palliative Care Network of Wisconsin. Retrieved September 24, 2021, from mypcnow.org/fast-fact/syndrome-of- imminent-death/

Worden, J. (2002). *Grief counseling and grief therapy*. Springer Publishing Co.

Zaner, R. (1988). *Death: Beyond whole-brain criteria*. Kluwer Academic Publishers.

8

GRIEF

Objectives

1 Define types of grief
2 Describe the stages of grief
3 Understand loss
4 Differentiate between bereavement and mourning

Grief is a complex, multifaceted reaction to loss. It affects relationships, both professional and personal. Experienced by all, grief reveals itself uniquely, individually, and culturally. Death is taboo. Discussing it makes people uncomfortable.

There is no rule book on how to grieve. Grief terminology can be confusing if not foreign. Different types of grief are mediated by circumstances. They include anticipatory grief, acute grief, and complicated grief (Rando, 1996).

Anticipatory grief is initiated with a grave or terminal diagnosis. The griever absorbs and adapts to the eventual finality of loss. This provides time for Patient, Family, and Clinician to complete "tasks of dying" and address "unfinished business." These tasks include repairing broken relationships, saying "goodbyes," and expressing what needs to be said.

Acute grief occurs immediately after the death of a loved one. It involves a separation response and a stress response. Shear (2015) observes that the symptoms of acute grief include physiological changes, such as variations in heart rate or blood pressure, sleep disturbances, and alterations to the immune system. These can lead to increased risk for diseases like myocardial infarction, Takotsubo cardiomyopathy, mood disorders, anxiety, and substance abuse.

Complicated grief diminishes ability to function to the point of "being stuck." Although the intensity of normal grief tends to lessen over time, complicated grief persists and blocks adaptation. Thoughts of the deceased and reminders of the loss

DOI: 10.4324/9781003257219-11

cause severe emotion and yearning (Horowitz et al., 1997). Often misdiagnosed, complicated grief must be distinguished from major depression and post-traumatic stress disorder (Shear, 2015).

Grief is the process of recognizing, expressing, and adapting to loss (Worden, 2002). There is no right or wrong way to grieve. The expression of grieving is individual and personal. We grieve because we care. There are many definitions of grief in scholarly, spiritual, and psychological literature. These disciplines agree that grief and its symptoms have no *rules* for behaving or feeling.

An individual's response to loss, including traditions, religious beliefs, and self-expectations, mediates the process and degree of grieving. Behaviors such as hysteria, aggression, fainting, total withdrawal, and denial may be present. Conversely, the opposite may be evident, such as shedding a single tear, quiet resignation, efficiency of tasks regarding the loss, or continuation of daily tasks without any indication of distress.

Grief takes time. Though grief modifies over time, it never completely goes away. The grieving process is lifelong, albeit without the same intensity and frequency of expression. Grief cannot be hurried, manipulated, or medicated. It can be delayed or postponed, but not indefinitely. Using a roller coaster metaphor, once you get on, you cannot get off. You may suspend the ride, but like the law of gravity, grief has its own progression. The grief "roller coaster" never ends. It continues through life with diminishing turns, drops, and speed. There is no escaping the need to grieve, and, like a roller coaster, grief has different stages.

Stages of Grief

Thanatologists, death educators, describe five common stages of grief: denial, anger, depression, bargaining, and acceptance. The stages are not necessarily experienced sequentially. By its very nature, grief is chaotic.

Shock/Denial is the first stage of grief. With a devastating diagnosis or an exacerbation, shock, disbelief, and confusion cause suspension of realistic thought. The brain struggles to absorb the "bad news." Patient and family members exhibit different behaviors ranging from numbness and resignation, quiet or hysterical crying, or screaming and/or physically aggressive actions.

Denial is a self-protective mechanism allowing the Mind time to process devastating information. It is the brain's way of marshalling resources in the face of inconceivable loss. Critical decisions are made while the griever is experiencing numbness and shock. The ability to function remains marginally intact while total comprehension and memory of events may be impaired.

BOX 8.1   JACQUELINE

Denial can interfere with memory of details. Information may be blocked. The griever is unable to see the evidence in front of them.

> *Jacqueline, a trained grief counselor, got the dreaded phone call from the ER. Her son had been in a car accident. Upon arrival, her 14-year-old son, Michael, was declared brain dead by a team of neurologists. The parent's, Jacqueline and Peter, first decision was to donate their son's organs.*
>
> *Per her training, Jacqueline began taking care of others. She prepared her three surviving sons and their friends for family visitations, funeral rituals, and the burial. Jacqueline organized her professional colleagues to help Michael's peer group. Throughout, she was efficient, thoughtful, and in total control. Describing her actions as an "out of body" experience, Jacqueline had little memory of the details of events following Michael's death.*

Jacqueline's denial and training as a grief counselor enabled her to take care of others. Distracted from the reality of her loss, she maintained her role as an expert. Her "out of body" experience was the coping mechanism, allowing her to function within the Relational System.

Anger experienced in grief has many sources. It is a response to loss. Helplessness leads to the frustration in the inability to "fix." Fear and anxiety contribute to anger. Displaced anger, a normal grief reaction, is defined as that which is inappropriately expressed toward others or self (Worden, 2002).

BOX 8.2   RUTH

Most Clinicians have experienced or witnessed agitation, anxiety, and anger expressed when giving bad news.

> *Ruth was referred to an ENT practice for evaluation of a persistent sore throat. After several trials of antibiotics and steroids, her primary care physician was puzzled by her lack of improvement.*
>
> *The specialists' exam revealed a large, ulcerated lesion of her left tonsil with ipsilateral neck nodes. Hearing the diagnosis of metastatic squamous cell carcinoma, Ruth protested that she had no history of alcohol or tobacco use. Her preacher husband immediately attacked the competence of the Clinicians. He rejected any and all treatment options including referral to other specialists.*
>
> *As the preacher became louder and more aggressive, his wife/patient became more withdrawn and visibly smaller. He shoved the physician aside to exit the exam room as his wife began to cry.*

The husband's anger was external and aggressive while his wife withdrew in fear. Both were expressing grief but in different ways.

Depression is a significant mood change, common in those who have suffered loss. Extremes in sleep, appetite, and energy may be evident in the same person at different times. The depressed person is highly distractible, feels isolated, and may become anxious. Treating situational depression with a prescription is ill-advised. As a normal grief reaction, this must be experienced. Medicating grief only delays the process.

Bargaining is an attempt to change the outcome of "bad news." Promising changes in personal behaviors, bargaining tries to control an uncontrollable situation with "would a," "could a," "should a"'s. Mixed with guilt and anger, this stage can become pathologic if not addressed and resolved. Bargaining is not always present as a stage of grief.

Acceptance is the stage of grieving where accommodation with loss occurs. The emotions and feelings regarding the loss stabilize. Grieving is adapted and integrated into normal daily living. Acceptance is a transient state. It is a temporary respite from the chaos of grief.

Loss

An inevitable part of life, loss is the basis of grief. It shapes us as we grieve. Personal losses begin at birth, leaving the protection of mother's womb. As the child matures, independence demands decreased reliance on the security of home. The process of aging itself is a series of losses. The older we become, the more we lose. Each loss is grieved uniquely.

Death is commonly referred to as loss. In reality, loss begins with diagnosis. Medical treatment, even if successful, incurs multiple losses for the Patient and their Family. Loss has aspects, as shown in Table 8.1.

TABLE 8.1 Aspects of Loss

Type of Loss	Characteristics of Loss
Physical	Change in physical capability, body image, loss of privacy
Mental	Confusion, anxiety, intellectual compromise (from medication and/or disease)
Social	Changing roles, friendships, finances, communities
Spiritual	Faith crises, questioning purpose and value of life

Physical Loss

A Patient's loss begins with the initial symptom of disease or trauma, when they recognize the absence of good health. They identify a physical abnormality and seek care. Consciously and formally relinquishing control, the Patient signs the admission forms. Their privacy is destroyed as every aspect of their lives may be examined to determine the etiology and extent of disease. Even control of the most private bodily functions is ceded as Clinicians demand samples of excretions, secretions, blood, and tissue. Access to their Body is unlimited and, on a time-frame not of the Patient's choosing (Pellegrino, 2006). Some Patients relinquish all decision-making, believing that the "doctor knows best." They may not get out of bed unless ordered. The concept of having control of one's own Body is lost.

Families experience loss with physical symptoms of sleep disturbance, appetite changes, and general malaise. There may be increased risk of new onset disease or exacerbation of chronic disease states. The stress generated by loss causes a physical response. Researchers have shown that Takotsubo cardiomyopathy is caused by an impaired ability to process and regulate emotions (Khalid, et al., 2018). Broken heart syndrome is a common phenomenon with spouses dying within days or months of each other.

Clinicians may have similar physical symptoms as Families. However, these may be more subtle or suppressed. Compassion fatigue and burnout syndrome results from unacknowledged grief over Patient losses (Engler-Gross et al., 2019). Demanding workloads, combined with maintaining a professional demeanor, may delay attention to grieving loss. The clinical tendency to ignore or self-medicate exacerbates the problem. Compassion fatigue and burnout will result from not processing loss.

Social Loss

Self-image changes with loss. It identifies the perception of a person's place and role in society. As losses are grieved, multiple factors influence and modify different aspects of an individual. For example, when losing a spouse, identity is changed from a "we" to an "I."

Losing one's healthy identity changes multiple roles. The father cannot function as "Dad." The caregiver is being cared *for*. The child is transformed from favored youth to primary caregiver. Friendships strengthen or dissolve. The severity and longevity of the disease process determine the magnitude of the roles' shift.

Financial status changes established roles for everyone. There is loss of income for the Patient and the caregiver and/or the cost of a caregiver. Care expenses encompass more than bills for treatment and services. Changes in living arrangements, health aides for disability, even dietary requirements can increase costs not covered by insurance.

There is a ripple effect from the Patient to Family to society. Unable to work, the Patient's absence impacts the workplace. Family life is redefined as job demands, and social interactions accommodate new priorities. As Family priorities change due to loss, the ripple effect expands and vacant roles must be filled by others. Social scarring varies in severity, affecting each member of the Patient's community. The Patient may not be able to return to roles in their Family and community as before.

An obvious example of roles shifting due to illness is illustrated by the SARS CoV-2 (COVID 19) pandemic in 2020. The entire world practiced "social distancing" – an unfamiliar role-changing social structure. The virus quickly caused

Patients to become critically ill. The surge in Patients resulted in shortages of ED and ICU beds, personnel, ventilators, and basic supplies.

Clinicians designed, manufactured, and recycled their own personal protective equipment. Workloads changed as many practices switched to telemedicine. Some specialties closed completely leaving providers unemployed. Other providers shifted to "hot spots" or different practices.

Clinicians lost colleagues from self-quarantine and/or the disease itself. As providers became Patients, they were treated, sometimes intubated, by co-workers. With each Clinician lost (permanently or temporarily), the gap was filled with clinical strangers, disrupting well-established teams.

Mental Loss

The loss of Patient's mental function is multifactorial. Physiological causes range from direct brain trauma to decreased oxygenation or electrolyte imbalances. Medications, not just anti-psychotics or opioids, can alter mental status. Isolation and sleep deprivation may contribute to psychosis. Addition or elimination of drugs, changes to routines, and social interactions cause disorientation. The Patient may be unable to understand the progress of his/her disease or the rationale for treatment.

Brains literally "shut down" as the Patient's perception is altered and unable to "reset." The Patient's confusion may precipitate behaviors including aggression, anger, crying, depression, hysteria, isolation, noncompliance, and withdrawal.

Clinicians are necessarily affected by these behaviors. Although they may appear unmoved, even aloof, they are invested. As professionals, Clinicians are expected to manage both the medical presentation and the surrounding environment. They must "control the room."

BOX 8.3 PATTI

Responding to Patients and Families adds to Clinician's own mental distress. By delaying self-care, Clinicians risk compassion fatigue and burnout.

Patti had seen Mitch numerous times as an inpatient. With right-sided heart failure, he frequently required hospitalizations for respiratory distress. Mitch was a gentle soul, calling all females "baby," no matter their age. He was thankful for his care and never complained.

Patti had just put in another 10-hour day as a hospitalist. Walking down the hallway, she met Cindy, a respiratory therapist. Cindy just weaned Mitch to BiPAP while he awaited hospice. He had signed a DNR.

There was no question that Patti needed to say goodbye to Mitch. Unable to summon the courage, she stepped into the hospital elevator and rode it up and down for 10 minutes. She then went to Mitch's room.

As mentioned before, "professional demeanor" is a distancing mechanism which protects the Clinician from personal attachments and the pain of loss. But in Patient/Clinician relationships, friendships develop.

Compartmentalizing feelings may be critical in time of crisis. However, the need for processing feelings must not be denied or suppressed. Unattended grief damages the Clinician's Spirit. Patti needed to say her "goodbyes" to Mitch for her own health and well-being. This completed her "unfinished business."

> *Entering Mitch's room, Patti quickly realized he was barely conscious. She pulled up a chair and sat next to him. As Mitch drifted in and out, he made eye contact with her and moaned, "How am I gonna tell them?" referring to his large family. Patti grabbed his hand and assured him he would find the words. Together, they shed silent tears.*

Allowing herself time to grieve gave Patti the strength to visit Mitch. She was "present" to him, more as a friend than a Clinician. Patti helped Mitch say his goodbyes. Care of the Personal and the Relational Systems is not an either/or issue. Both must be attended to.

Spiritual Loss

Spirituality gives meaning to life. "Why me?" is an expected response to debilitating, grave, and terminal diagnoses. Loss attacks everyone's established moral balance and value systems. "Bad news" disrupts one's moral compass.

According to Kubler-Ross (1969), spiritual suffering evolves from the perception of disease as divine punishment. Catastrophic illness or trauma may foster a spiritual crisis. Feelings of guilt can cloud understanding of the medical circumstances.

Modern medicine has very little experience in aiding and comforting suffering. Chaplains are attached to hospitals. However, rarely do Clinicians consult them for their Patients or themselves. It is not part of traditional medical training. In general, a Patient's spiritual care is addressed only as part of formal palliative or hospice consult.

Many Patients believe their suffering has redemptive quality. Suffering can be seen as atonement for wrongs committed during a person's life. As the Patient struggles to understand and adapt to the disease process, sheer fatigue, and grieving multiple losses diminish spiritual strength.

"Spiritual maturity" gives meaning to losses incurred in suffering. Dr. Bernie Seigel observes that some patients describe their disease as a "gift." "That doesn't mean they don't wish to be well, but they wouldn't give up what they have achieved because of their illness" (Siegel, 1989).

Spiritual growth and maturity correlate to pain tolerance, attitude, and compliance with treatments (Veatch, 2009). As the individual struggles for meaning and purpose, losses are defined and grieved. The resulting scar strengthens spiritual foundation.

Families feel helpless. In many cases, they pray for a cure and/or an end to suffering. Families with strong connections tend to weather crises better than those without spiritual support (Puchalski, 2006). Sometimes, Families and friends become discouraged because they did not get their prayers "answered." They may feel guilt or anger, feeling responsible for the Patient's suffering.

Children grieve differently than adults. Each age level and milestone cause a new grieving period as the child grows into greater comprehension of their loss. Their re-grieving will stabilize in adulthood. Younger children may experience abandonment issues and/or regression. Physical ailments, hyperactivity, poor appetite, outbursts of anger, and sleep disturbances are common in all age groups.

Science and spirituality exist with tension. Acknowledging spiritual loss may be anathema to the scientifically focused. However, Clinicians ignoring their spiritual element create an unhealthy balance. Spiritual loss must be recognized and grieved.

Loss has many faces. Clinicians often refer to a cure as a "return to baseline." However, the return to health is the creation of a new baseline, the new "normal." Every disease process or trauma creates scars – physical, mental, and spiritual. The idea that a patient is "as good as new" is incorrect and unrealistic.

Bereavement and Mourning

Bereavement and mourning are frequently used interchangeably, but they are distinctly different. Bereavement is a normal reaction to an abnormal loss. It refers to the period of grief and mourning after death. The length of bereavement is influenced by how close the individual was to the deceased, or whether the death was expected. Bereaving the "year of firsts" describes initial experiences surviving holidays, birthdays, anniversaries, etc. without the deceased. Identity changes from spouse to widow, child to orphan, etc.

Mourning refers to coping behaviors that are used to accommodate loss. Surviving loss includes completing tasks of mourning. Worden (2002) and Rando (1996) describe these tasks of mourning as:

1   Accepting the reality of the loss
2   Working through the pain of grieving
3   Adjusting to an environment in which the deceased is missing
4   Maintaining connections with the deceased while establishing a new identity

Funeral rituals are heavily influenced by culture, religion, region, and tradition. Some indigenous tribes expose the Body to the elements. Jewish religion requires burial within 24 hours. In northern regions, burials are delayed until the ground thaws. Internment in aboveground mausoleums may be required in areas subject to flooding. Other traditions include funeral pyres or cremation. Wakes or visitations may be somber remembrances or raucous celebrations.

Grief has no time limit. Reorganizing life around loss is a daunting personal task requiring energy and focus – two qualities diminished by grief. The loss of a loved one is permanent. Living with that loss continues as necessary accommodations are made and adjustments transform daily life. As the tasks of mourning are completed, living is redefined. There is no "closure" that ends grief. Closure is the sense or experience of successfully living with a significant loss which can only be personally defined.

Relational Care and Grief

With Relational Care, attention is paid to the Patient, Family, and Clinician's grieving process – individually *and* relationally. Initially, when a Patient receives a terminal diagnosis, there may be crying, confusion, or stoicism. These reactions are only a part of what is happening with the Patient. Internally, Body, Mind, and Spirit are trying to make sense of chaos, as illustrated in the Personal System (see Venn diagram 2.1). At the same time, the Patient is relationally experiencing how the Family and Clinician are reacting in grief.

There may be physiological, emotional, and psychological grief reactions that the Patient hides. The Patient may want to protect and comfort their Family. In relationship with their Clinician, the Patient may respond in a manner that "mirrors" the Clinician's demeanor.

When given bad news, Families respond as if they understand, even if they do not. They need time to absorb information as they protect and comfort their sick relative. Shock has many faces; clarity is not one of them.

Clinicians need to grieve losses encountered in practice. They are not expected to explore the degree and depth of their Patients' losses. However, recognition and appreciation of loss improve the Patient/Family/Clinician relationships.

Being aware is important to self-care. Pressing duties may require a delay, but grief cannot be safely ignored or compartmentalized indefinitely. Most clinical programs have limited training in loss and grief. What there is does not address self-care (Skistrom et al., 2019).

Intense focus on the Body blinds Clinicians to other elements of care. Without training, Clinicians tend to cope poorly (Skistrom et al., 2019). Clinicians train to make quick decisions in a crisis, while putting their emotional response on hold. Dealing with delayed emotions is not addressed. The consequence of unresolved grief is cumulative. Damage to the Clinical Mind and Spirit will eventually impact the Clinical Body. Professional and personal relationships suffer.

BOX 8.4   SEMINAR FOR MENTAL HEALTH THERAPISTS

In a seminar for mental health therapists, a description of Clinicians' training, both now and in the past, was outlined. The tendency to treat death as the result of an error, or ignoring it entirely, was described. When the therapists heard that many Clinicians never grieve a Patient death, one observed, "No wonder most of my practice is doctors' families!"

The Venn diagrams (Figures 2.1 and 2.2) show the interface of physical, mental, and spiritual elements within Personhood. In the Relational System, Patient, Family, and Clinician create and maintain connections as the function of the Healthcare Collaboration. Loss changes that connection. The relationship adapts and remains.

Questions for Reflection

1   Complete the Personal Loss History found in Appendix B.2. What was surprising about your responses?
2   How do *you* grieve the loss of a Patient?

References

Engler-Gross, A., Goldzweig, G., Hasson-Ohayon, I., Laor-Maayany, R., & Braun, M. (2019). Grief over patients, compassion fatigue, and the role of social acknowledgement among psycho-oncologists. *Supportive Care in Cancer, 28*, 2025–2031. https://doi.org/10.1007/s00520-019-05009-3

Horowitz, M., Siegel, B., Holen, A., Bonanno, G., Milbrath, C., & Stinson, C. (1997). Diagnostic criteria for complicated grief. *American Journal of Psychiatry, 154*, 904–910.

Khalid, S., Khalid, A., & Maroo, P. (2018). Risk factors and management of Takotsubo cardiomyopathy. *Cureus. 10*(5), e2626. doi: 10.7759/cureus.2626

Kubler-Ross, E. (1969). *On death and dying*. Scribner.

Pellegrino, E. (2006). Toward a reconstruction of medical morality. *American Journal of Bioethics, 6*(2), 65–71. https://doi.org/10/1080/15265160500508601

Puchalski, C. (2006). *A time for listening and caring*. Oxford University Press.

Rando, T. (1996). Complications in mourning traumatic death. In K. Doka (Ed.), *Living with grief after sudden loss: Suicide, homicide, accident, heart attack, stroke* (pp. 139–159). Hospice Foundation of America.

Shear, K. (2015). Complicated grief. *The New England Journal of Medicine, 372*(2), 153–159. https://doi.org/10/1056/NEJMcp1315618

Siegel, B. (1989). *Peace, love, and healing.* Harper and Row.

Skistrom, L., Saikaly, R., Ferguson, G., Mosher, P., Bonato, S., & Soklaridis, S. (2019). Being there: A scoping review of grief support training in medical education. *PLoS ONE, 14*(11), e0224325. https://doi.org/10.1371/journal.pone.0224325

Veatch, R. (2009). *Patient, heal thyself.* Oxford University Press.

Worden, J. (2002). *Grief counseling and grief therapy.* Springer.

9

CAUTIONARY ISSUES

Objectives

1   Define countertransference
2   Differentiate care of special populations
3   Recognize the importance of language and culture

Introduction

Certain medical encounters require special attention because they are "outside of the box." Cautionary issues affect the Patient's disease course outside of standardized treatment protocols.

For example, Takotsubo cardiomyopathy is directly related to stress levels. The Patient presents with unstable angina. The cause of their chest pain is NOT atherosclerotic heart disease but an aberrant neurological response to stress (Khalid et al., 2018). Relational Care enables the Clinician to recognize and navigate cautionary issues. "One size fits all" has no place in clinical practice.

Countertransference is bias that changes the Clinician/Patient relationship. Usually an unconscious experience, training is needed to avoid it.

BOX 9.1   JENNIE

The awareness that countertransference exists is the first step in managing it.

Jennie's grandmother suffered from Alzheimer's for years. As a child, her grandmother spent months in her home. Once she required nursing home

---

DOI: 10.4324/9781003257219-12

> *care, Jennie never saw her grandmother again. As a Physician Assistant, Jennie's responsibilities included nursing home rounds. There, she bonded inordinately with one particular resident. Over time, Jennie identified the smell of the patient's hand lotion as her grandmother's favorite. The distinctive perfume brought bittersweet memories of time spent with her grandmother. Recognizing countertransference, Jennie was able to normalize her interactions with her Patient.*
>
> Jennie's increased time spent with the resident was a natural reaction, resulting in a change in her Clinical behavior. Once recognized, Jennie managed her interactions appropriately.

Countertransference may be conscious or unconscious, in either or both Patient and Clinician. Triggered by dynamics or events, countertransference is "a natural, appropriate, and inevitable emotional response" (Johnson & Katz, 2006, p. 4).

Reflection and awareness are necessary to manage countertransference. A wide range of emotions influence the Patient/Clinician relationship. "If we cannot engage a patient around his or her belief system because of our reaction to their beliefs, we have allowed countertransference to adversely affect our care for this person" (Wendleton et al., 2006, p. 29).

There is extensive evidence showing the correlation between physical disease and mental health (Ohrnberger et al., 2017). Clinicians have little, if any, exposure to mental health diagnosis and treatment strategies (Nymberg et al., 2000). Many practitioners are uncomfortable with assessing mental health needs of a Patient or Family. Yet, the awareness and use of mental health referrals are limited.

Some large practices have integrated mental and physical health care. Reduced insurance compensation for mental health services discourages the majority of medical practices from adopting this policy (Kaplan, 2014). Many qualified mental health specialists resort to fee for service because of difficult and limited insurance compensation.

Special Populations

Age differences, language difficulties, cultural misunderstanding, and Clinical "red flags" necessitate special consideration.

Caring for children is different from caring for adults. Their values need to be respected without treating them as "little adults." Children are difficult because of countertransference issues. No one wants a sick or injured child. It triggers a visceral response connected to personal experience. This countertransference interferes with clinical objectivity.

Pediatric Clinicians are trained and understand the basic rules in interacting with children.

Rule 1: Never try to hide the truth from children. They do not need to know every detail of a diagnosis, either for themselves or for their loved ones. However, their fertile imaginations will generate far worse scenarios than reality.

Rule 2: Children are masters at observing and interpreting clues. They are proficient in detecting body language, tidbits of conversation, and masked emotions. However, children are unable to interpret the information correctly or completely.

Rule 3: Children know something is wrong. They are sensitive to voice tone or looks. Their reality is based on their creative assumptions and "magical thinking." Their "data" influence flawed interpretations.

BOX 9.2 TOMMY

Children are master spies with limited reasoning.

> John and Mary's 11-year-old son, Tommy, battled leukemia for several years. The last round of chemotherapy proved ineffective. Tommy would die soon. Both parents grieved and struggled with how to tell him. They turned to pediatric palliative care for help. The doctor agreed to a family conference.
>
> The doctor began by summarizing Tommy's treatment to date. She explained the latest results as he listened intently. Tommy glanced repeatedly back and forth between his weeping parents and his doctor. Finally, he asked, "Is that all?!"

Tommy overheard his parents' emotional discussions behind closed doors. He feared his worst-case scenario, a divorce. To Tommy, his death was no surprise; he already knew and accepted it on his level. His family remaining together was invaluable to him.

Our children are supposed to outlive us. A child's death creates a physical, emotional, and spiritual grief greater than the loss of a spouse. It is a loss so devastating that statistics show the majority of marriages do not survive the death of a child (Shrank et al., 2005). The loss of a child is the loss of the future.

Schonfeld and Quackenbush (2009) describe how children grieve differently than adults. As the child matures, they will re-grieve the loss at their new level of understanding. This process will continue to adulthood.

In infancy, there is no real comprehension of death. However, infants may react as if they have been abandoned. They are sensitive to the distress of the Family and the disruption of routines.

By the age of 2, the child, with limited expressive language, may verbalize "dead" without any understanding. They may refer to a deceased pet as "no more" or "gone."

At the age of 3–4, "magical thinking" conceptualizes death as temporary. The child expects the loved one to return. Simple language appropriate for the child's development is necessary. The explanation that "the Body has stopped working and will not start again" requires repetition in many different ways, many times over. In their immature understanding, preschool children may experience grief with a sense of guilt. They believe their "bad" behavior contributed to the loss of their loved ones.

Preschool and young school-aged children may demonstrate "clingy" behavior. They may revert to bedwetting, sleep problems, and fears of another loved one dying. School disruptions and somatic complaints may surface.

Six- to nine-year-old children understand death is irreversible and final to the extent of their maturity. They spend a lot of time thinking and asking questions about life and death. This age can believe their thoughts, actions, or emotions can cause harm to others.

Preadolescents (aged 8–12 years) have an adult understanding of death. However, they have not yet learned to identify and deal with feelings. They may develop a fascination with death, expressing interest in both the physical process of dying and the rites and ceremonies surrounding death.

Older children and teens may focus on schoolwork, sports or hobbies, and socializing with their peers. They do not like to be alone. Adolescents may try to "step up" into the gap left by the deceased and assume their responsibilities. Previous routines, friendships, and interactions with others assist in adjusting to life with loss. The successful outcome of a child experiencing loss rests primarily on having at least one significant adult for love and guidance. Children's grief groups and counselors are helpful in the process of their grieving. Local hospice facilities maintain referral lists.

Elders (65 years of age or older) are the largest cohort of the general population (Mather et al., 2015). Healthier and living longer, seniors contribute to the workforce and economy far longer than their predecessors. Despite multiple comorbidities, they are becoming disabled at a later age. Conversely, disabled elders' healthcare cost is skyrocketing. "By 2030, health care spending will increase by 25%, largely because the population will be older" (CDC, 2013, p. 5).

The "silver tsunami" has the potential to be a financial disaster. As seniors live longer, their health care and supportive needs are draining resources (personal, governmental, and institutional) at alarming rates. The majority of nursing home residents (60–70%) require long-term care because of some form of dementia (Robnett & Chop, 2015).

Although our aging population is exploding, the number of gerontologists is shrinking (Robnett & Chop, 2015). While Gawande (2014) believes this is due to the economics of gerontology, there are other factors involved. Geriatric practice requires expertise in chronic care, critical care, and drug interactions. A confusing diagnostic picture becomes a balancing act of choosing the lessor of evils.

BOX 9.3 RICK

Rick had been a PA in neurology for over 15 years. In his practice, he cared for numerous dementia patients and was experienced and adept at addressing concerns. Andrea (67) brought in Arty (74), her husband of 47 years, for his regular appointment. Arty was diagnosed with Alzheimer's Disease over 7 years ago. Medication was effective in slowing the rate of decline. Today's testing showed worsening symptoms.

As Rick chatted with the couple, Andrea asked for directions to the restroom. After directing her, Rick returned to the exam room to find Arty in tears. He immediately sat down and asked Arty what was wrong. "I'm so alone! I am so afraid and alone. I don't know who that person is that brought me here. I know she is nice to me, but I don't know who she is!"

Rick had seen dementia patients who did not recognize loved ones. Usually, it did not cause them this much distress. Rick was at a loss. As he gently tried to calm Arty down, Rick asked if there was anything he could do to help. Arty, drying his tears, replied, "Just don't tell her. She is so nice. I don't want to upset her. I'm so very tired of being all alone."

When recounting this story to his team, Rick teared up. He felt empathy and helplessness at the same time. His compassion allowed him to be present to Arty. This eased suffering in both.

Elders live alone, with family members, in assisted living, or nursing homes. Cognitive decline exacerbates the stress on Patient and Family. Requiring support, seniors may "rotate" through multiple households in different locations. A demented Patient relies on the familiarity of a set environment and routine. Medical and/or socioeconomic factors create disorienting changes. This can accelerate cognitive decline. The elder's role in society has shifted from wise advisor and historian of tradition, to economic drain and familial liability.

Encouraging seniors to make their preferences known is critical. Advance Directives help Clinicians and Families make difficult decisions, honoring the Patient's value system. Using a document such as "The Five Wishes" (Appendix B.10) facilitates necessary conversations in a simple, clear, and comprehensive manner. These conversations need to occur *before* crisis or change in mental status.

The LGBT community presents challenges in both mental and physical health. Language and cultural sensitivity are necessary to build trust. A safe environment begins with awareness, training, and communication.

The LGBT community has become more visible in society after generations of hiding. Research shows this population is less likely to have appropriate medical care (Lombardi, 2001). Patient comfort is only one block to adequate healthcare. "Barriers . . . include negative healthcare experiences and beliefs" (Gruskin, 1999, p. 5). Insufficient financing, lack of trained Clinicians, and blatant and/or subtle discrimination exacerbate an already tenuous relationship.

BOX 9.4   KIM

Training in the appropriate language, approach, and care of the LGBT population is necessary throughout clinical education.

> *Standardized Patient (SP) events are patient actors displaying a specific set of complaints and symptoms for students in a more realistic setting. The encounters are monitored and filmed. A valuable tool for sensitivity and exposure to LGBT patients takes place in a safe, instructive environment. Kim, a medical student, entered the room and started the interview.*

Kim: *"Hi, Mrs. Smith. My name is, Kim. What brought you to the clinic today?"*
Mrs. Smith: *"My wife made me come in because she says I snore."*
> *Kim glanced quickly at her paper, confirming the SP was portraying a female patient. "You said your wife?"*
Mrs. Smith: *"Yes, that's right, my wife."*
Kim: *"But . . . you're . . . female. And you have a wife?!"*
> *Kim was stunned and unable to proceed. She was called out of the room and counseled by her instructor. Kim was given time to process the experience. Starting over, she conducted herself in a professional manner.*

Bias exists. It is often subconscious. Tools are available to promote self-awareness of biases. The Harvard Implicit Bias Test is a free website and ongoing study. It can be found in Appendix B.3.

LGBT health concerns include depression, increased use of alcohol and other drugs, sexual abuse, and hate violence. Patient comfort is promoted in the initial interaction with staff. With the first phone call, enquiring about preferred pronouns and sexual identity is HIPAA compliant and trust building. Birth gender, sexual preferences, and gender identification become part of the clinical assessment.

Special Needs populations include physical, mental, and social disabilities. Myriad in number, they require additional resources outside of normal clinical tools. This text is incapable of addressing them all. A thorough history and physical, including a mental status exam and caregiver assessment, gives more information of special needs. Incorporating the appropriate specialist(s) into the interdisciplinary team improves overall care. Open collegial consultation needs to be the norm rather than the exception.

Language

Misunderstanding and/or miscommunication are often a result of problems with language. Gender, culture, ethnicity, tradition, socioeconomic status, experience, and education influence it. Verbal and nonverbal, regional dialects, jargon, and slang contribute to different interpretations. It is vitally important to verify that intended meaning is communicated. Incongruence occurs when language and intention are mismatched. It is demonstrated by inconsistency of words and body language. Congruence is necessary for legitimate Informed Consent.

Informed Consent MUST be on the patient's level and in a language they understand (American Medical Association Ethics, 2021). "Medicalese" is not appropriate unless the Patient is a Clinician and is comfortable with that language.

BOX 9.5 JACKSON

In this case study, the doctor communicated in highly accented "medicalese," while his body communicated competency and confidence. Consequently, the Patient signed the Informed Consent without understanding.

> The surgical resident, JC, was a star in the OR. He was hampered by a significant Chinese accent. As a first-generation immigrant, even the staff had difficulty understanding some of his orders. One Friday evening, he was called to the ER to see a gunshot victim. Jackson, a middle-aged, inner city, southern male, listened intently as JC gave him the clinical synopsis. This included the textbook description of an open exploration of the abdomen, an ileostomy, with a "takedown" re-anastomosis at a later date. Jackson agreed to the procedure, signed the Informed Consent, and JC left to write orders for the OR.
>
> The Physician Assistant, Asher, stayed with Jackson. As she locked eyes with him, she softly asked, "Do you understand what is about to happen?" Jackson confessed that although he had signed Informed Consent, he had not understood a word that JC had said. Using hand drawn pictures and simpler language, Asher described the surgery again to the visibly relieved patient.

Asher recognized fear, doubt, and confusion in Jackson's body language. Using different tools of simpler language and drawings, she explained the procedure again. Only then, the Patient verbally and nonverbally communicated congruence.

Communication aids include translators, visual images, models, and pencil and paper. Another common strategy ensuring understanding is "teach-back." This technique has the Patient restate, in their own language, the Clinician's information. Teach-back is effective for Family members, providing clarity within the Healthcare Collaboration.

Culture

Cultural norms strongly influence the Healthcare Collaboration. Individuals, Families, and/or communities manifest their cultures through their preferences. Expressed by beliefs, language, dress, food, and rituals, Families are the experts on their own culture. Ethnic, employment, socioeconomic, age, and national cultures determine how we live and die. Respecting, appreciating, and honoring cultural influences are necessary for clear communication.

Each culture has different value systems. However, sometimes the cultures are difficult to define. Students receive education on various ethnic cultures (Caucasian, African American, Asian, Hispanic, etc.). However, practitioners may not realize that each Family, individual, and relationship has its own particular culture.

Families make decisions reflective of their traditions and experiences. For example, the Family culture may favor the patriarch as the final decision-maker. Stoicism may fit a Family's mores. Religious rituals support Patient and Families. The possibility and uniqueness of cultural expression are limitless.

Studies delineate various culture groups' beliefs regarding end of life (Shrank et al., 2005). African Americans have a high distrust of medical systems and the authority figures within. Family support, family values, and religious influences play a greater role in decision-making. Quality of life is not as important as longevity. African Americans are strongly supportive and open to Spiritual discussions.

Caucasians value quality of life as influenced by financial and legal concerns. Interestingly, they are split regarding open discussion of Spirituality and Spiritual concerns by Clinicians.

Asian culture values patriarchy. The eldest male is responsible for making the decisions for the Family. They honor and revere their elders and ancestors. Self-sacrifice preserves the Family unit.

BOX 9.6 MRS. CHEN

In Asian cultures, the individual is not as important as Family.

Mrs. Chen was brought to the ED by two of her daughters and her teenage granddaughter, who served as the translator for the group. Mrs. Chen was first-generation Chinese, having lived in the United States for years. She had a few phrases and a handful of English words. Mrs. Chen gave her history through her granddaughter. The two non-English-speaking daughters added additional information.

Mrs. Chen, a widow, spent every morning in the family's grocery store. She was working there when she became dizzy and passed out. Through her translator, she vehemently denied additional symptoms. Her daughters reported that Mrs. Chen appeared to have lost weight and was fatigued more than usual. When this was communicated, Mrs. Chen denied the reported symptoms. When pressed, she grudgingly admitted she had some unexplained weight loss.

Diagnostic studies revealed the cause of her symptoms. Mrs. Chen had a large colorectal tumor, threatening to occlude her descending colon. This was causing her anemia and weight loss. Despite the size of the mass, her team concluded there was no metastatic disease. An aggressive excision of the mass followed by chemoradiation would give Mrs. Chen the best chance of a cure.

The multidisciplinary team needed to tell Mrs. Chen about this complex plan. However, whenever the discussion was initiated, she would interrupt the Clinicians, stating, "No! Talk to son, talk to son!" Even with the granddaughter interpreter, Mrs. Chen emphatically refused to listen. Conceding defeat, the team agreed to a meeting with the son, the family, and the hospital translator.

Even with everyone present, Mrs. Chen appeared to be disinterested. The Clinicians described the diagnosis and proposed treatment. The translator confessed the Chen family's dialect was unfamiliar to her. She believed the son understood the message.

The Family requested time with Mrs. Chen to explain what would happen. A weekend pass from the hospital was issued. Mrs. Chen signed out. Despite telephone calls, letters, and telegraphs, she and the family were never seen again.

The surgeons were reluctant to proceed with a surgery that required an extensive procedure. A colostomy and port placement for chemotherapy required Mrs. Chen's full understanding. Subsequent chemoradiation required compliance despite risks and side effects. There was no assurance the son was fully capable and willing to explain to his mother. The team believed Mrs. Chen competent to sign Informed Consent. Her son's signature on the forms would not be acceptable.

Western medicolegal culture clashed with the Family's culture, rendering the Healthcare Collaboration ineffective. There was a question of secondary gain. This takes place when another benefits through illness or incapacitation of someone. The son could use his mother's illness to gain more control of the family business. Communication in the Chen family was chaotic at best. Communication among Patient, Family, and Clinicians was worse.

Clinician Conflict

Medicine is its own culture with its own language, mores, and rituals (protocols). Within this culture are specialties, and the training is universal and individual simultaneously. Different points of view regarding patient care occur and can cause conflict. How differences are resolved is important to the successful functioning of the multidisciplinary teams.

The goal of multidisciplinary teams (MDTs) is to reduce medical errors and increase Patient safety through communication, team collaboration, trust, and respect. MDTs are more effective in healthcare than a single provider approach and are common in practices today. Most Clinicians are familiar with and serve on multidisciplinary teams, but the full effectiveness of the team is rarely realized (Lin et al., 2018).

Clinicians communicate through reports, orders, and notes. Training in peer-to-peer communication, team leadership, and conflict resolution is lacking. Barriers to the success of MDTs include limited time, territorialism, hierarchy, and lack of understanding of team members' skill set and experience. For example, studies show that nurses advocate Patient preferences, whereas advanced providers focus on the biomedical data of the case (Lamb et al., 2011).

BOX 9.7   WHEN CLINICIANS FORGET THE PATIENT CENTERED APPROACH

An old joke illustrates the problems that arise when Clinicians forget the patient centered approach:

> *An internist, oncologist, and nephrologist were coordinating care of an elderly man with multiple comorbidities including COPD, leukemia, and end-stage renal disease. The internist let the rest of the team know that the patient was dying. He would not be alive much longer. That afternoon, the oncologist heard from the floor nurse that the patient had died. He continued his rounds but then thought, "Maybe one last round of chemo can be obtained so the autopsy will show tumor regression." He loaded up a round of chemo and went down to the morgue. Finding the patient's storage drawer, he opened it to find an empty bed with a note reading, "In dialysis" with the date, time, and nephrologist's signature.*

In the fight against the disease, sometimes the Patient, and their preferences, are lost.

MDTs are Patient-centered without the Patient in attendance. Families are not consulted unless the MDPOA is required in a decision.

Mutual respect and trust, equality, conflict resolution, constructive discussion, absence of personal agendas, and the ability to ask questions and obtain clarification are facilitated through good communication (Soukup et al., 2018). Relational Care provides tools to avoid or resolve conflict by using specific language that defuses what could develop into team dysfunction (see Chapter 13). Respecting colleagues' input is vital.

Impaired Providers

Defined as the "inability or impending inability to practice according to accepted standards as a result of substance use, abuse, or dependency" (Baldisseri, 2007, p. 106), impaired providers are a danger to their Patients, their colleagues, and themselves. Studies have shown that healthcare providers have similar rates of substance abuse as the general population. Certain specialties have an increased representation in substance abuse surveys. Psychiatry, anesthesiology, and emergency medicine, in that order, are at higher risk for abuse (Baldisseri, 2007).

More providers use substances without meeting the criteria for abuse or dependence. The rate of substance use in medical providers is five times higher than in the general population. More clinicians are *users* but not *abusers* to the point of addiction.

Chemical dependency is multifactorial. Causes include neurobiological, genetic, psychological, personality, and occupational factors. These occupational factors include stress, access, attitude, and exposure. Providers believe their medical knowledge allows control, protecting them from addiction. This behavior has been termed "professional invincibility" by the Center for Alcohol and Addiction Studies (Kenna & Lewis, 2008).

Diana Quinlan (1995) in her paper on impaired providers states that dependency does not present with a single sign or symptom. Gradual changes in behavior take place over time. Notable behaviors associated with chemical dependency include mood swings, frequent tardiness or absenteeism, increasing difficulty with co-workers and supervisors, and deterioration of work performance (see Appendix B.4). Colleagues of impaired providers frequently enable their substandard behavior. Covering for the impaired providers' lapses and ignoring signs of dependency is common (see Appendix B.5).

Integration

In healthcare, as in life, nothing is perfect. Relational Care appropriately guides the Healthcare Collaboration with informed decisions. Awareness of cautionary issues compels the search for solutions. Providers are not required to have all the answers. Addressing issues openly and asking for help demonstrates care and support for all members. Unconventional strategies and untraditional resources create solutions for care.

Questions for Reflection

1   Informed Consent, whether assumed, verbal, or written, is a legal requirement before administering treatment. How do you know your Patient truly understands their options?
2   Have you ever suspected a co-worker of being impaired? What is your legal/ ethical obligation to them and Patients?

References

American Medical Association Ethics. Code of medical ethics opinion 2.1.1 informed consent. *Principles of Medical Ethics: I, II, V, VIII. (2021).* www.ama-assn.org/delivering-care/ ethics/informed-consent

Baldisseri, M. R. (2007, February 23). The impaired healthcare professional. *Critical Medicine,* (2 Supplement), S106–S116. https://doi.org.10.1097/01/CCM.0000252918.87746.96.

Center for Disease Control (2013). *The state of aging & health in America 2013.* cdc.gov/ aging/pdf/state-aging-health-in-america-2013.pdf

Gawande, A. (2014). *Being mortal: Medicine and what matters in the end.* Metropolitan Books.

Gruskin, E. P. (1999). *Treating lesbians and bisexual women.* SAGE Publications.

Johnson, T., & Katz, R. (2006). *When professionals weep.* Taylor and Francis Group.

Kaplan, G. (2014). *Total recovery.* Rodale Press.

Kenna, G., & Lewis, D. (2008). Risk factors for alcohol and other drug use by healthcare professionals. *Substance Abuse Treatment and Policy, 3*(3). https://doi.org/10.1186/1747-597X3-3

Khalid, S., Khalid, A., & Maroo, P. (2018). Risk factors and management of takotsubo cardiomyopathy. *Cureus, 10*(5), e2626. https://doi.org/10/7759/cureus.2626

Lamb, B.W, Allchorne, P., Sevdalis, N., Vincent, C., & Green, J. (2011). The role of the cancer nurse in the urology multidisciplinary team meeting. *International Journal of Urologic Nursing, 5,* 59–64. https://doi.org/10.1111/j.1749-771X.2011.01119.x

Lin, W., Sun, J., Chang, S., Tsai, T., Wu, P., Huang, W., Tsao, C., & Lin, C. (2018). Effectiveness of the multidisciplinary team model in treating colorectal cancer. *Gastroenterology Nursing, 41*(6), 491–496. https//doi.org/10.1097/SGA.0000000000000348

Lombardi, E. (2001). Enhancing transgender health care. *American Journal of Public Health, 91*(6), 869–872. https://doi.org/10.2105/ajph.91.6.869

Mather, M., Jacobsen, L., & Pollard, K. (2015). Population bulletin: Aging in the United States. *Population Reference Bureau, 70*(2). www.prb.org

Nymberg, J., Selby, J., Fernandez, C., & Grimsley, D. (2000). The art of quietly making noise: Orchestrating the integration of behavioral healthcare into a multispecialty medical group. *Families, Systems, & Health, 18*(10), 105–121. https://doi.org/10.1037/ h0091856

Ohrnberger, J., Fichera, E., & Sutton, M. (2017). The relationship between physical and mental health: A mediation analysis. *Social Science and Medicine, 195,* 42–49. https://doi. org/10.1016/j.socscimed.2017.11.008

Quinlan, D. (1995). The impaired anesthesia provider: The manager's role. *American Association of Nurse Anesthetists, 63*(6).

Robnett, R., & Chop, W. (2015). *Gerontology for the health care professional.* Jones and Bartlett Learning.

Schonfeld, D., & Quackenbush, M. (2009). *After a loved one dies- helping children grieve.* New York Life Foundation.

Shrank, W., Kutner, J., Richardson, T., Mularski, R., Fischer, S., & Kagawa-Singer, M. (2005). Focus group findings about the influence of culture on communication preferences in end of life care. *Journal of General Internal Medicine, 20*, 703–709. https://doi.org/10.1111/j.1525-1497.2005.0151.x

Soukup, T., Lamb, B., Arora, S., Darzi, A., Sevdalis, N., & Green, J. (2018). Successful strategies in implementing a multidisciplinary team working in the care of patients with cancer: An overview and synthesis of the available literature. *Journal of Multidisciplinary Healthcare,* Dove Medical Press, *11,* 49–61. https://doi.org/10.2147/JMDH.S117945

Wendleton, D., Johnson, T., & Katz, R. (2006). Caregiving of the soul: Spirituality at the end of life. In T. Johnson & R. Katz (Eds.), *When professionals weep* (p. 29). Taylor and Francis Group.

10

STRESS, COMPASSION FATIGUE, AND BURNOUT

Objectives

1   Describe stress
2   Differentiate between compassion fatigue and burnout
3   Understand moral distress

Introduction

Stress is necessary to life and is present all the time. In today's general psychology, the term stress is synonymous with negative influences (Le Fevre et al., 2006). Conversely, positive stress, *eustress*, fosters creativity, productivity, and imagination. Too much stress, known as *distress*, negatively affects physical health and well-being. Hans Selye defines stress as "a non-specific response of the body to a demand" (Szabo et al., 2012, p. 472). He describes the Body's reaction to stress in three stages: 1) alarm, 2) resistance, and 3) exhaustion. Distress symptoms are found in Compassion Fatigue and Burnout. Resilience mitigates the damage.

Clinicians displaying changes in attitude toward Patients, Families, and peers may be demonstrating the first signs of Compassion Fatigue (CF) and Burnout Syndrome (BOS). When a provider dreads their workplace and has diminished enthusiasm, energy, and gratification, CF may be the cause and/or the effect. Colleagues may be the first to recognize behavioral changes. As symptoms intensify and multiply, physical, emotional, and spiritual damage may develop.

CF and BOS are debilitating and sometimes career ending. They may co-occur without a specific sequence (Mattioli et al., 2018). Often a byproduct of Secondary Traumatization Syndrome (STS), early recognition and intervention can prevent CF and BOS.

DOI: 10.4324/9781003257219-13

CF and BOS affect all healthcare providers. In 2018, the Canadian Medical Association's survey of physicians revealed a 30% rate of BOS with 8% suicidal ideation within that year (Rozario, 2019). Numerous studies indicate that BOS is high in specific specialties with rising numbers and severity. Certain specialties – anesthesia, psychiatry, general practice, and general surgery – are at higher risk (Dutheil et al., 2019). The meta-analysis indicated an increase of cases in women. Despite good preventative care, both CF and BOS are persistent risks.

Definitions

Stress is often misunderstood. We need stress to function. The medical definition of stress is a Body's reaction to any change that requires an adjustment or response (Szabo, et al.). Stress is a normal reaction to everyday pressures. Problems arise when stress impacts day-to-day functioning.

Most Clinicians thrive on stress. Emergency situations stimulate an addictive adrenaline rush. Healthcare providers enjoy the challenge and pace of work up to a point. Challenge stress or eustress is defined as overcoming problems through teamwork, innovation, effort, and skill (Kim & Beehr, 2020).

BOX 10.1   TONY

Tony, a head and neck oncologist, and Regina, his Physician Assistant, were performing a laryngectomy with neck dissection. As the case progressed, Regina had to pause her first assist duties to manage an inpatient issue on the floor. Upon her return, as she reintegrated into the procedure, Tony remarked, "You know, OR is my happy place. I don't have to worry about the phone, the office, home, nothing except what's right here in front of me. Life gets simple in the OR. It's just us against the cancer."

Although the case was extended and stressful, it was perceived manageable by the team.

However, as the pace of work and bureaucratic demands increase, occupational stress rises. Occupational stress, hindrance demands, or distress describe the reaction to unmanageable obstacles that thwart progress (Kim & Beehr, 2020). High levels of stress are described physically as feeling tense, restless, nervous, or worried, with disturbed sleep from stressful thoughts (Almen et al., 2020).

Resilience is the ability to "cope with stress and vital to stay in balance" (Vinkers et al., 2020, pp. 12–16). Psychologists have identified characteristics that increase it. Positive attitude, optimism, accepting failure as a form of learning and feedback, and the ability to regulate emotions help develop resilience.

Two decades later, there is still no accepted definition of compassion fatigue. Researchers describe CF as "work-related stress response in healthcare providers that is considered a 'cost of caring' and a key contributor to the loss of compassion in healthcare." This meta-analysis also described CF as "a state in which compassionate energy expended surpasses the restorative process provided by compassion satisfaction, resulting in a loss of the power to recover." This phenomenon leads to "intrusive empathetic strain" and patient avoidance (Sinclair et al., 2017, pp. 9–24).

Charles Figley (1995) first described Compassion Fatigue (CF) as associated with the reduction in empathy for the client/patient. Prior to 1990, CF applied to the frustration of charitable group volunteers. Today, CF is seen as a significant risk factor for healthcare professionals.

Physical symptoms of CF include exhaustion, insomnia, headaches, abdominal pain, etc. (Sinclair et al., 2017). Behavioral symptoms include loss of satisfaction, emotional exhaustion, cynicism, self-centeredness, and a sense of not being oneself (Henson, 2020). CF is characterized by a change in attitude with sudden onset.

Sometimes linked with secondary traumatic stress and vicarious traumatization, compassion fatigue is insidious and stealthy in its progression (Sansbury et al., 2015). Work, once satisfying and fulfilling, becomes burdensome and annoying. Attitudes become linked with negative and positive treatment outcomes. Competency may not be diminished but satisfaction is.

Long-term outcomes (Mattioli et al., 2018) are described as increased risk for physical illness, rage, apathy, depression, insomnia, weight gain or loss, and trouble with concentration and memory. The decrease in energy and dissatisfaction is similar to depression and Burnout. If not treated, CF can lead to both.

BOX 10.2   CARLOS

Healthcare professionals are generally unaware of how CF develops. The sudden onset of diminished empathy can be overwhelming.

Susan, a PA hospitalist, had known Carlos, a Hispanic construction worker, for less than a year. She was surprised to see him back on her patient list with a severely low platelet count. With a previous diagnosis of chronic idiopathic thrombocytopenia, the 24-year-old had been admitted for an elective splenectomy late in the fall. Carlos was a very compliant patient and pleasant to work with, despite his inability to speak English. He recovered as his platelet count responded. Carlos was discharged without any complications.

Months later, Carlos' platelet count was again alarmingly low. He returned to the hospital for transfusion and further evaluation by specialists not available in his indigent clinic.

Hematology recommended a pulse of high-dose corticosteroids. Although Carlos' platelet count responded, he developed a cough with fever. His CXR revealed a surprising "whiteout." Pulmonologists subsequently performed a diagnostic and therapeutic bronchoscopy.

The findings were devastating. Carlos had a fungal infection. The steroids allowed the infection to flourish. Therapy for the fungal infection required him to be off corticosteroids. Consultants believed the fungal infection was causing the ITP. Corticosteroids necessary to stop his bleeding blocked the antifungal agent. It was a Catch 22.

Over the course of several weeks, Carlos declined. He required mechanical ventilator support for fungal pneumonia as his ITP worsened. Carlos' once strong healthy body became bloated and grotesque. Carlos and his wife, Juanita, were devout Catholics. She filled his room with pictures of saints and candles. Juanita arranged for a special blessing by their priest.

Susan began to come earlier to the ICU, switching her routine so that Carlos' unit was the first visit in her schedule. Part of her knew she was avoiding Juanita and their two children.

Susan was on Carlos' old medical floor when she was paged. Carlos' team had received permission from Juanita to take him off the ventilator. The intensivist did not expect him to live longer than a few minutes without the mechanical support.

As she hung up the phone, Susan leaned her forehead against the wall and stated to Casey, the case manager, "That's it. I'm done. I can't do this anymore."

When Casey heard that Carlos was being withdrawn from life support, she made Susan sit down. Upon hearing that Susan had not eaten for over 5 hours, she urged her to eat something. "I can't. I feel sick. I don't want anything." Susan remained hunched in Casey's chair with her eyes closed and her head down. Casey went into the patient pantry and brought back a brownie and a carton of milk. "Here, eat this." she commanded. "I can't. I don't want it. I just can't." "Then sit there until you DO eat it. I'll be back in a minute. You have to take at least one bite before I get back." Casey responded.

It took time, but Susan was able to choke down the brownie and milk. Casey checked to make sure she had finished everything. Then she asked, "Feel better?" "I guess." Susan responded. "Good" Casey replied, "Now go get 'em, tiger."

As Carlos' Body declined, Susan was physically affected. She began her days earlier to avoid seeing Juanita. She worked harder, slept poorly, and skipped meals.

Susan's countertransference, identifying with Juanita and her two children, impacted her ability to interact with the Family. Susan felt guilt when she saw the children, so close in age to her youngest child.

Juanita cared for Carlos in her own way. The importance of the priests' blessings and religious objects (pictures of saints, crosses, and candles) were necessary for Carlos' spiritual care despite normal ICU restrictions. As a South American Catholic, Juanita kept a previously lit candle under the bed near Carlos' head. Nursing and housekeeping respected her belief (culture) this helped "light Carlos' way to heaven."

Healthcare providers are trained in triaging care, including their own grief. Casey delayed her grieving to care for Susan. She recognized that Susan was overwhelmed by CF. Casey provided necessary urgent care.

The Healthcare Collaboration responds, adapts, and attends for each element within its Relational System. Body, Mind, and Spirit were challenged by Carlos' disease progression. Typically, spiritual symbols and priests' blessings are discouraged in ICUs. By making an exception, the staff cared for both Carlos and Juanita.

With the devastating diagnosis of Carlos' fungal infection, Susan's Personal System suffered. She was unable to recognize, much less mediate, her CF. Casey identified Susan's distress and appropriately intervened. In this scenario, the Healthcare Collaboration functioned with a devastating loss.

Some might question if Susan was suffering from Burnout Syndrome (BOS). BOS is described as a "state of mental weariness" (Schaufeli & Bakker, 2004, p. 293). Although similar to CF in presentation, BOS happens over time. It appears as changes in personality, perspective, and behavior (Henson, 2020). CF is a "natural response" resulting from Patient/Clinician interactions, while BOS results from Patient/Clinician interactions *and/or* Clinician/managerial interactions (Mattioli et al., 2018). Table 10.1 summarizes characteristics of CF and BOS.

The 11th Revision of the International Classification of Diseases (ICD-11) defines burnout as a syndrome resulting from chronic workplace stress. It is characterized by exhaustion, personal and professional distancing, negative feelings regarding the job, and reduction in performance (World Health Organization, 2019). Physiological symptoms of burnout include sleep interruption, social withdrawal,

TABLE 10.1 Comparison of Compassion Fatigue and Burnout Syndrome (Henson, 2020)

Compassion Fatigue	Burnout
Sudden onset	Develops over time
Emotional and physical exhaustion	Emotional exhaustion
Change in Patient interaction	Change in Patient and/or Managerial interaction
Apathy	Cynicism
Helplessness	Hopelessness
Desensitization to Patients and Families	Desensitization to everything and everyone
Depersonalization *for* Patients	Depersonalization *of* others

poor judgment, and cynicism. BOS has been associated with depression, anxiety, drug and alcohol abuse, deterioration in health, and poor patient outcomes Worrisome psychological symptoms may be marked by perfectionism, pessimism, the need for control, and reluctance to delegate.

Lifestyle contributors, such as not taking care of Body, Mind, and Spirit, lack of social support, and the inability to seek peer feedback, increase the danger of burnout. Studies indicate that BOS is more prevalent in those of younger age, female gender, unmarried status, and difficult working conditions (Kesarwani et al., 2020).

Sleep deprivation, use of unhealthy coping mechanisms (i.e., drug or alcohol use), failure to maintain a work–life balance, and negative self-assessment increase the risk of BOS. Additional factors are an unbalanced load of bureaucratic tasks, insufficient compensation, electronic health record inefficiency, difficult patients, and difficult employers. The Maslach Burnout Inventory, see Appendix B.8, is a self-assessment tool to determine the risk of burnout.

Without intervention, blunted emotions with hopelessness and helplessness lead to Major Depression, even suicidal ideation (Kesarwani et al., 2020). Self-medication by Clinicians, using prescriptive or illegal drugs or alcohol, exacerbates the problem. An unclear Mind with a narrowed perspective is unable to recognize the need for help or realize what options are available (Dissanaike, 2016).

Neither CF nor BOS can be discussed without mentioning the impact of the Coronavirus 19 pandemic in 2020. Initially seen in Wuhan, China, in December 2019, the pandemic swept through the world stressing healthcare systems and providers past the breaking point. There are numerous instances of providers being forced to utilize scoring methods (APACHE III and SOFA) to triage patients for scarce ventilators and medications. Rationing of resources violated the core bioethics of Clinicians.

Clinicians themselves contracted the virus. Their recovery or demise forced once well-coordinated teams to dissolve and reorganize. The numbers of Patients requiring critical care literally overwhelmed facilities.

Unsurprisingly, the rate of depression and anxiety rose. In Wuhan, China, 12.7% of healthcare workers had depression symptoms and 20.1% had debilitating anxiety (Du et al., 2020). A prominent US Emergency Department physician and department head, Dr. Lorna Breen, committed suicide in the spring of 2020, after contracting the virus. Her family stated that Dr. Breen returned to work 10 days after being diagnosed. Just before her death, she described the "onslaught of patients" that overwhelmed her department.

BOX 10.3 COMPASSION FATIGUE

Interviews with New York City healthcare providers revealed the toll taken by COVID-19. On April 24, 2020, Julianne Nicole, an ICU nurse, posted on Facebook her experience with one of her COVID-19 patients, a 23-year-old male.

> *"I was destroyed by his clinical course in a way that has only happened a few times in my nursing career. It wasn't his presentation. I've seen that before. It wasn't his complications. I've seen that too. It was the grief. It was his parents. The grief I witnessed yesterday, was the grief that I haven't allowed myself to recognize since this runaway train got rolling here in early March. I could sense it. It was lingering in the periphery of my mind, but yesterday something in me gave way, and that grief rushed in . . . First it was our normal white body bags. Then orange disaster bags. Then blue tarp bags. We ran out of those too. Now, black bags."*
>
> In the face of this pandemic, compassion fatigue and burnout syndrome occurred. It was so fast and widespread; it was difficult, if not impossible to prevent. The city did its best with demonstrations of support. But the toll on both Clinicians and caregivers was significant.

Caring for victims of trauma can result in secondary traumatization which can lead to Secondary Traumatic Stress Disorder (STSD). STSD is due to "indirect exposure in a professional context" (Jacobs et al., 2019, p. 1). While not experiencing the traumatic event directly, the aftermath of injury, for example, dismemberment, disfigurement, disability, and death, can cause reactions in the caregiver that require attention. Similar in symptomology to Post–Traumatic Stress Disorder (PTSD), victims experience recurring thoughts, flashbacks of the initial impacts of exposure, depression, anxiety, and isolation. The frequency and intensity of these symptoms may not be as great as experiencing full-onset PTSD.

In Appendix B.7, the Secondary Traumatic Stress Scale (STS) measures responses over a 7-day period. When scored, the scale concentrates on three symptomatic behaviors: Intrusion, Avoidance, and Arousal. The Impact of Event Scale is another screening tool for PTSD found in Appendix B.9, measuring the same behaviors.

Post–Traumatic Stress Disorder (PTSD) can be a consequence of secondary traumatization in healthcare. PTSD was first documented in veterans but has since been seen in emergency workers, victims of trauma and sexual assault, healthcare workers, and others. The symptoms of PTSD include a psychological re-experiencing of a specific trauma. Common behavioral symptoms are flashbacks, avoidance behavior, and increased arousal and agitation (Sendler et al., 2016). Four specific environments are likely to trigger PTSD: working in conflict zones, residency training, treating trauma patients, and practicing medicine in rural areas.

In 2010, a systematic review of studies regarding the prevalence of PTSD in institutionalized healthcare workers revealed PTSD symptoms in 8–29% of surveyed providers (Robertson & Perry, 2010). One striking finding was the lower response rate of less than 50% from participants. Nursing respondents reported higher scores than doctors. Additionally, physicians were found to be less likely to report or seek treatment for PTSD.

The classic definition of moral distress is a psychological trauma when one witnesses a trusted individual/leader committing atrocities. It occurs when the individual is unable to prevent or stop actions that violate their moral beliefs and ethics. Moral distress in medicine is caused by Clinicians experiencing guilt or distress at their perceived inability to provide adequate healthcare (Rozario, 2019).

The COVID pandemic is causing many providers to leave their professions. Triage, because of scarce resources and overwhelming patient numbers, exacerbates the frustration, exhaustion, and helplessness. While not always found in cases of compassion fatigue and burnout, poor leadership and moral distress compound the issue.

Integration

Some Clinicians are better protected from Compassion Fatigue and Burnout Syndrome than others. Coping mechanisms include strong family life, social support, recreational activities, active self-care strategies, spiritual connectedness, and cognitive coping skills. Autonomy, positive leadership, and team cohesiveness are characteristics of a supportive work environment that promotes physical, mental, and spiritual health (Lee et al., 2013). All of these develop and support resilience. Chapter 13, Taking Care of the Caregiver, offers specific strategies for self-care.

Preventative training in stress management should begin in school and continue throughout healthcare careers. Skills in dealing with Patient death and addressing fears regarding safety in the workplace are necessary and should be readily available without consequence (Sendler et al., 2016). Quick screening techniques measuring stress alert supervisors and managers of the need for intervention (Thoresen et al., 2010).

The Healthcare Collaboration works when the elements of Patient, Family, and Clinician (Relational System) contribute to the health of the Personal System (Body, Mind, and Spirit). All members of the Relational System may experience compassion fatigue and burnout. Prevention and timely intervention within an interactive Healthcare Collaboration provides an agile response in critical times.

BOX 10.4   SANDY

Healing takes place for all – often outside of standard clinical protocols.

Sandy, a vibrant, beautiful 17-year-old, returned to the OR for the third time. Diagnosed at 14 with thyroid cancer, she had a recurrence successfully excised over a year ago. Her screening PET scan this month showed increased activity along her left anterior cervical chain. The team felt confident that the "heat" on the PET scan was increased activity from scarring, but it still warranted a look.

There was very little tissue left after a total thyroidectomy and a second, left anterior neck dissection for positive nodes. Scarring from previous surgeries and radioactive iodine therapies made a relatively simple case difficult and tedious. The regular landmarks were gone or buried in scar tissue. Bleeding was an issue; vessels were friable from the radiation.

When pathology called with the frozen section results, the call was refused because of intricate work. Once the repairs had been completed, the surgeon, Jason, and his PA, Avery, were able to look at the handwritten note from pathology. Sandy had three small nodes enmeshed within the sample tissue. Each was about the size of a grain of rice, and all were positive for recurrent cancer.

At the crushing news, the room fell silent. Jason dropped his hands onto the field and lowered his head. He sadly stated, "That's it. If she has another recurrence, she'll require external beam radiation. She'll be scarred for life. We can't do anything more here." The entire team was paralyzed with grief, and a few sniffles were heard.

Avery broke one of the first rules of surgery she'd ever been taught. She reached across the table and grabbed Jason's hands. "You know what we're going to do now? We're going to lay hands on Sandy and pray. And you're going to lead us." Jason was well known for praying for and with his cancer patients. The entire team, without being asked and without any regard to religious preferences, laid both hands on some part of Sandy's body. Jason led them in a prayer for her healing and they resumed the operation without further comment or complications.

In the OR, Sandy's Body was healed. Avery's break in protocol facilitated healing of the entire team's Body, Mind, and Spirit.

Two years later, both Jason and Avery received invitations to Sandy's high school graduation party. Avery thought about the invitation and called Sandy's mother, Evelyn.

"Evelyn, I'm calling about this wonderful invitation. And I really appreciate the thought behind it. I don't know what Jason is going to do, but I won't be able to attend and I want to tell you why. If for any reason, we have to operate on Sandy again, I won't be able to do a good job. I can be casual friends with you, but I just can't be that close to Sandy and be a good PA for her. I hope you understand."

Establishing boundaries benefited the entire Healthcare Collaboration – Patient, Family, and *Clinician*.

Questions for Reflection

1   What is your favorite way to decompress after a stressful week? When did you last take time to decompress?
2   Complete the Professional Quality of Life Measure (ProQOL) found in Appendix B.6. This tool indicates compassion fatigue, burnout, secondary traumatization, and post-traumatic stress disorder.
3   Complete the Maslach Burnout Inventory. The link is found in Appendix B.9. Were you surprised by your score? What are you going to do about it?

References

Almen, N., Lissperes, J., Ost, G. T., & Sundin, O. (2020). Behavioral stress recovery management intervention for people with high levels of perceived stress: A randomized controlled trial. *International Journal of Stress Management, 27*(2), 183–194. https://doi.org/10.1037/str0000140

Bride, B., Robinson, M., Yegidis, B., & Figley, C. (2004). Development and validation of the Secondary Traumatic Stress Scale. *Research on Social Work Practice, 14,* 27–35. https://doi.org/10/1177/1049731503254106

Dissanaike, S. (2016). How to prevent burnout (maybe). *American Journal of Surgery, 212*(6), 1251–1255. https://doi.org/10/1016/j.amjsurg.2016.08.022

Du, J., Dong, L., Wang, T., Rao, C., Fu, R., Zhang, L., Liu, B., Zhang, M., Yin, Y., Qin, J., Bouey, J., Zhao, M., & Li, X. (2020). Psychological symptoms among frontline healthcare workers during COVID 19 outbreak in Wuhan. *General Hospital Psychiatry, 67,* 144–145. https://doi.org/10.1016/j.genhosppsych.2020.03.011

Dutheil, F., Aubert, C., Pereira, B., Dambrun, M., Moustafa, F., Mermillod, M., Baker, J., Trousselard, M., Lesage, F., & Navel, V. (2019). Suicide among physicians and healthcare workers: A systematic review and meta-analysis. *PLoS ONE, 14*(12), e0226361. https://doi.org/10.1371/journal.pone.0226361

Figley, C. R. (1995). Compassion fatigue as secondary traumatic stress disorder: An overview. In C. R. Figley (Ed.), *Compassion fatigue: Coping with secondary traumatic stress disorder in those who treat the traumatized* (pp. 1–20). Routledge.

Henson, S. (2020). Burnout or compassion fatigue: A comparison of concepts. *Medsurg Nursing, 29*(2), 77–95.

Jacobs, I., Charmillot, M., Solech, C., & Horsch, A. (2019). Validity, reliability, and factor structure of secondary stress scale – French version. *Frontiers in Psychiatry, 10,* 191. https://doi.org/10.3389/fpsyt.2019.00191

Kesarwani, V., Husaain, Z., & George, G. (2020). Prevalence and factors associated with burnout among healthcare professionals in India: A systemic review and meta-analysis. *Indian Journal of Psychological Medicine, 42*(2), 108–115.

Kim, M., & Beehr, T. (2020). Thriving on demand: Challenging work results in employee flourishing through appraisals and resources. *International Journal of Stress Management, 27*(2), 111–125. https://doi.org/10/1037/str0000135

Lee, R. T., Seo, B., Hladkyj, S. Lovell, B. L., & Schwarzmann, L. (2013). Correlates of physician burnout across regions and specialties: A meta-analysis. *Human Resource Health, 11,* 48. https://doi.org/10.1186/1478-4491-11-48

Le Fevre, M., Kolt, G., & Matheny, J. (2006). Eustress, distress and their interpretation in primary and secondary occupational stress management interventions: Which way first? *Journal of Managerial Psychology, 21*(6), 547–565.

Mattioli, D., Walters, L., & Cannon, E. (2018). Focusing on the caregiver: Compassion fatigue awareness and understanding. *Medsurg Nursing, 27*(5), 323–328.

Robertson, N., & Perry, A. (2010). Institutionally based health care workers' exposure to traumatogenic events: Systematic review of PTSD presentation. *Journal of Traumatic Stress, 23*(3), 417–420. https://doi.org/10.1002/jts.20537

Rozario, D. (2019). Burnout, resilience, and moral injury: How the wicked problems of health care defy solutions, yet require innovative strategies in the modern era. *Journal of Canadian Chiropractors, 62*(4), E6–E8. https://doi.org/10/1503/cjs.002819

Sansbury, B., Graves, K., & Scott, W. (2015). Managing traumatic stress responses among clinicians: Individual and organizational tools for self-care. *Trauma, 17*(2), 114–122. https://doi.org/10.1177/1460408614551978

Schaufeli, W. B., & Bakker, A. B. (2004). Job demands, job resources, and their relationship with burnout and engagement: A multi-sample study. *Journal of Organizational Behavior, 25*(3), 293–437. https://doi.org/10.1002/job.248

Sendler, D., Rutkowska, A., & Makara-Studzinska, M. (2016). Vol 30:4. How the exposure to trauma has hindered physicians' capacity to heal: Prevalence of PTSD among health-care workers. *The European Journal of Psychiatry, 30*(4).

Sinclair, S., Raffin-Bouchal, S., Venturato, L., Mijovic-Kondejewski, J., & Smith-Mac-Donald, L. (2017). Compassion fatigue: A meta-narrative review of the healthcare literature. *International Journal of Nursing Studies, 69*, 9–24. https://doi.org/10.1016/j.ijnurstu.2017.01.003

Stamm, B. H. (2016, January). *The secondary effects of helping others: A comprehensive bibliography of 2,017 scholarly publications using the terms compassion fatigue, compassion satisfaction, secondary traumatic stress, vicarious traumatization, vicarious transformation and ProQOL.* www.proqol.org.

Szabo, S., Tache, Y., & Somogyi, A. (2012). The legacy of Hans Selye and the origins of stress research: A retrospective 75 years after his landmark brief "Letter" to the Editor# of Nature. *Stress, 15*(5), 472–478.

Thoresen, S., Tambs, K., Hussain, A., Heir, T., Johansen, V., & Bisson, J. (2010). Brief measurement of posttraumatic stress reactions: Impact of Event Scale-6. *Society of Psychiatric Epidemiology, 45*, 405–412.

Vinkers, C., Van Amelsvoort, T., Bisson, J., Branchi, I., Cryan, J., Domschke, K., Howes, O., Manchia, M., Pinto, L., De Quervain, D., Schmidt, M., & Van der Wee, N. (2020). Stress resilience during the Coronavirus pandemic. *European Neuropsychopharmacology, 35*, 12–16. https://doi.org/10.1016/j.euroneuro.2020.05.003

World Health Organization. (2019). *Burn-out an "occupational phenomenon": International Classification of Diseases.* Retrieved September 16, 2021 from who.int/news/item/28-05-2019-burn-out-an-occupational-phenomenon-international-classification-of-diseases

PART IV
Creating Solutions

11

TELLING BAD NEWS

Objectives

1 Describe the Buckman/SPIKES Protocol
2 Understand the difference between Advance Directives and POLST

Introduction

Trained in medical protocols to diagnose and treat the Body, Clinicians rely on their knowledge and expertise. They respond quickly, competently, and efficiently to relieve pain and restore health. However, when health cannot be restored, delivering "bad news" is necessary. Put simply, Clinicians are ill prepared. They find the communication of bad news disconcerting.

Clinicians communicate with each other in half sentences, anacronyms, and slang buzzwords. Latin terminology describes the anatomy and diseases. Testing and evaluation use Space Age terms. Telling bad news requires a language of compassion and understanding. It is unfamiliar and uncomfortable to Clinicians.

Definition

Bad news is usually given with a diagnosis of a terminal disease process. These include a new chronic diagnosis, a significant unrecoverable decline, amputation, etc. Bad news does not affect the Body alone. It impacts the Mind and Spirit, causing extreme reactions. Patient and Family behaviors will range from complete cognitive shutdown to hysteria.

The Relational System experiences a shift as the Personal System reacts to the information. The Healthcare Collaboration is tasked with "What do we do next?" A time of confusion is commonplace as the bad news is realized and sinks in. Each

DOI: 10.4324/9781003257219-15

individual and the Personal and Relational Systems are changed. Roles shift as changes in behaviors and responses result. Adaptation occurs as each Body, Mind, and Spirit restores balance within Patient, Family, and Clinician.

Tools

Clinicians must be facilitators of successful communication. In obtaining a full history and physical, a social and family history is included, either directly or through a Patient completed form. With Relational Care, these valuable data are utilized rather than ignored. The process of gathering and reviewing this personal information reveals the communication style of the Patient. The clinical note has a specific format: Chief Complaint, History of Present Illness, Review of Systems, etc. It is incumbent that Clinicians observe the language of the Patient and Family. This develops and incorporates a common understanding of communication styles. Using appropriate language develops openness, trust, and compliance.

BOX 11.1 DREW

Drew had been a patient at Matt's clinic for years. He was a fairly healthy, 45-year-old IT support engineer who used Matt, a PA, as his provider. He also supervised the clinic's computer and phone systems. Drew was a more frequent visitor for clinic IT issues than for his health.

Matt had been tracking Drew's slowly rising blood pressure. It was time to start medication for better control. Knowing Drew's tendency to "forget" to complete prescribed courses of treatment, Matt knew he had to make an impression on the importance of compliance.

As Matt described Drew's blood pressure and the need for treatment, the expected glazed look began to appear. Matt quickly shifted into a mutual language. "Remember that virus update you installed for us earlier this year? How often does it update for us now?" "Of course." Drew replied, "It's the best we have. It updates hourly."

Matt nodded. "Yes, and that's exactly just like this drug. You need to take it every single day. It prevents your own hard drive, your brain, from corrupting. If you miss taking it, your computer is open to attack. Just like with the antivirus updates, if you don't take your medicine every day, you won't know there's a problem until it's too late."

Most Clinicians experience difficulty stressing compliance treating the "silent killer," hypertension. In order to ensure Drew's comprehension and compliance, Matt used language that Drew understood.

Using verbal language, including metaphors and analogies, promotes under-standing. Observation of Patient's physical response and engagement informs the depth of comprehension. Body language, like "tells" in poker, reveals the truth. Congruence occurs when body language, verbal language, and comprehension are "*in synch*." The importance of language is discussed in Chapter 9.

Many communication problems arise during End of Life (EOL). Patients, Fami-lies, and other caregivers expect Clinicians to know when and how to initiate conversations regarding EOL preferences. However, studies have shown that Clini-cians are not well trained or comfortable with this responsibility (Buckman, 1992). Additionally, Clinicians have difficulty in accurately prognosticating a Patient's survivability and/or demise (Luce & Rubenfeld, 2002). Subsequently, tools were developed to facilitate telling bad news. These tools, taught as a component of EOL care, belong in everyday clinical practice.

During crisis, Patient and Family become confused and distracted. They strug-gle to comprehend the medical diagnosis and treatment. Being aware of incongru-ence during critical discussions can prevent and mediate confusion and conflict. Cognizance and appreciation of each individual's perspective further support deci-sion-making. The Healthcare Collaboration is the consensus of the Patient, Family, and Clinician coming together to make the right choice, ranging from aggressive curative treatment to removal of life support.

The Joint Commission (JC) mandates assessment of the Patient's spiritual needs (2018). Often, this portion of the social history is either skipped or delegated to a Patient-completed form. Tools such as FICA and SPIRIT (Table 11.1) are dutifully memorized for boards and then forgotten in practice.

These assessments allow the Clinician to explore Patient values. They are NOT designed to be filled out as a standardized form or item checklist. The success of these tools, used in conversation, depends upon an already established relationship.

Knowing when to have these difficult, usually lengthy, conversations is a skill. A simple cold or minor trauma does not require full knowledge of Patients' values and wishes. With a change in a chronic condition or new disease onset, a review is indicated as soon as possible.

TABLE 11.1 Comparison of Spirituality Assessment Tools: FICA and SPIRIT (Borneman et al., 2010; Sulmasy, 2006)

FICA	SPIRIT
Faith, belief, meaning – religion and spirituality	Spiritual belief system
Importance and Influence of beliefs upon life	Personal spirituality
Community	Integration with a spiritual community
Address in care	Ritualized practices and restrictions
	Implications for medical care
	Terminal events planning

BOX 11.2 SARAH

A new major disease diagnosis or an acute exacerbation of a previously controlled, chronic ailment may be unexpected. Physician Assistants and Nurse Practitioners add valuable consultation time to Patient care. Specifically trained to educate, they facilitate communication within the Healthcare Collaboration.

> In her first year of clinical practice, a Physician Assistant was rounding on Sally. As the PA finished her exam, the attending physician entered the room. He quietly closed the door and leaned against the frame, crossing his arms over his chest. "I just talked to the radiologist about your results. I'm afraid your colon cancer has spread to your liver with multiple metastases. This is very bad news. It's why you're jaundiced. I'm ordering a hospice consult for you. Ms. Jenkins will finish up here and answer any of your questions."
>
> The attending left as both Sarah and the PA were literally stunned, unable to process the news. The PA reached out for Sarah's hand as she began to cry.

This encounter left the Healthcare Collaboration unbalanced and ignored. Patient and Clinician needs and values were not addressed. The Relational System was never reestablished.

In 1992, Dr. Robert Buckman published on how to tell bad news to patients. Known by the mnemonic SPIKES (Table 11.2) or Buckman Protocol, it was groundbreaking work. Addressing the poor communication between Clinicians and Patients, it was initially designed for EOL situations.

TABLE 11.2 The Buckman or SPIKES Protocol for Delivering Bad News to Patients (Buckman, 1992)

Step	Basics	Rules
Setting	In person, with the right people present, at the right time	Schedule enough time, take off the white coat, speak to the patient at eye level
Patient knowledge	Find out how much the patient knows about what is going on	Be sure to pay attention to verbal and nonverbal language
Information sharing	Find out how much the patient WANTS to know	Always give the option for additional information at a later date
Knowledge	Sharing information	Allow the patient to respond and process in their own time
Empathy	Identify and acknowledge patient's reaction	Be present: Do not be afraid to touch
Strategy	Plan for the future	Reassure the patient they are in control. Schedule follow-up meetings

In Relational Care, SPIKES is used in common, everyday practice as a communication and relationship tool. Integration of care, Relational Care, is not limited to end of life.

Dr. Buckman's SPIKES Protocol is summarized as follows:

Setting: Try to make the delivery of bad news in person and privately, if at all possible. This is more of a personal conversation than a clinical progress report. It is best that the Patient is aware that the Clinician needs to have a conversation with them. Significant others or close friends may need to be present or be asked to leave. Schedules for therapy and/or treatment may need to be rearranged. Staff needs to be alerted the Clinician will be unavailable. Removing the white coat and accouterments of medicine when entering the room alerts the Patient this is NOT a normal Patient/ Clinician encounter. Sit at eye level to give the impression that time is not an issue.

Patient Knowledge: Enquiring about the Patient and their plans for the day are common, open-ended questions to re-establish connection. Knowing how the Patient perceives their status is important. Asking about what the Patient knows of the current therapy and how it is making them feel is a good way to start. Understanding where they are generates the basis for the continuing conversation. To proceed to the next step, the Clinician needs to know what the Patient understands about their disease process and what the Patient expects.

Information Sharing (asking how much the Patient wants to know): Most Patients want to know what is happening to them. Some want to know every detail of medical information. Most just want basic data – will they live, will they have pain, how long will they have to stay in the hospital, etc. Ascertaining what level of understanding the Patient wants is difficult for most Clinicians. The urge to retreat into medical jargon and repetition of data must be resisted. Patients want and deserve simple, understandable facts.

Knowledge Sharing: Patients need to be prepared to receive bad news. Clinicians need time and observation to best deliver it. The Clinician should clearly and distinctly outline the diagnosis, treatment plan, prognosis, and support available. The description of bad news should be as simple and free of "medicalese" as possible. During this portion of the conversation, it is important to check the Patient and Family members' understanding of the message. Being sensitive to verbal *and* body language reveals information overload, fatigue, and emotional stress. Most Patients are aware that something has changed for the worse. Honesty by "naming the beast" is necessary. It brings transparency by exposing the uncertainty and fear. Using proper terminology gives a measure of control to the Healthcare Collaboration.

Empathy: Empathy is not just acknowledging another's feelings. It is giving permission to express them. Clinical training stresses a stoic, academic distancing from Patients. This is inappropriate when giving bad news. Although the Clinician is still providing care, the disease is in control. The sensitivity of recognizing the grief of the Patient, Family, *and* Clinician is therapeutic for all. Touch is not only allowed. It is encouraged.

BOX 11.3 MAX

Hugs and expressions of gratitude are common as the Patient finally has formal "permission" to feel bad and/or stop pretending for Family and caregivers.

Max was walking down the hallway when he was intercepted by his supervising physician. Dr. Johns was infuriated. Max was surprised and puzzled. "Explain this to me!" Dr. Johns whispered, in barely controlled rage. "I operate on them. I give them more time with their families. But you are the one who gets the hugs!" Max remained confused until Dr. Johns described he had witnessed one of their terminal cancer patients hugging and thanking Max before their appointment with the surgeon.

The source of Dr. Johns' anger was not from Max's incompetence. The surgeon was reacting to the lack of affection from the Patient. Max's Relational Care for his Patient resulted in a strong personal bond.

Support: Everyone is afraid of dying alone. Despite advances in public education, hospice and palliative care have poor reputations in certain Patient populations. Many Patients view hospice as a place where they "let you die alone" or that it is a warehouse for dead and dying. One suggestion in broaching this topic in a less threatening way is to introduce hospice as a "ramp up" of care. In other words, additional personnel and therapies will be added to the regimen to improve Patient comfort.

To combat the Patient's fear of abandonment, the plan, particularly follow-up, is critical. The plan should include appropriate referrals to hospice/palliative care, continuing and/or modifying therapies, and reviewing Advance Directives. Equally important, increased comfort care and stratification of goals need to be discussed and implemented. Rather than diminished care, Patients will typically experience an increase in care options. Most Patients are relieved to have control. They are fully in charge of what happens next. Stress relief is so great; many Patients experience physiological as well as psychological improvement.

Dr. Bernie Seigel describes the impact of bad news delivered gracefully to Patients (1998). A terminal diagnosis gives the Patient knowledge, permission, and time to prepare for dying. They may complete a "bucket list," heal relationships, say goodbye, and/or put their lives in order. These tasks relieve relational, psychological, and emotional pain and suffering. It offers a measure of control in an uncontrollable situation.

Advance Directives (AD) are formalized statements of the Patient's preferences near the end of life. Up to 76% of Patients facing EOL will be unable to participate in their care decisions (Motely, 2013). The AMA supports and encourages early discussions regarding Advance Directives. There are different forms of varying complexity. Written by hospitals, government agencies, and nonprofit organizations, there are forms specific for age groups and educational levels.

Five Wishes, published by Aging with Dignity (2021), is a document addressing EOL preferences for adults (see Appendix B.10). Available in 30 languages, it is legally valid in most states. *Voicing My Choices* is written for seriously ill adolescents and young adults, aged 11–18 years. It meets the legal requirements for AD in most states. *My Wishes* is a version developed for children, completed by parents, and is not legally binding. All three documents are written simply, avoiding medical and legal jargon.

Early in the history of ADs, there were essentially only two choices – full code status or Do Not Resuscitate (DNR). Those choices have now grown into a myriad of options for personalization of care. Patients can choose aggressive treatment (full code status), partial treatment (IVs, feeding tubes, ventilation, etc.), Allow Natural Death (comfort care only), or DNR (no intervention at all). ADs can be specific or generic. They may be changed at any time and as often as the Patient wants.

POLST is a portable medical order set for Patients who are seriously ill or with advanced frailty. The form is designed to be completed by the Clinician, in conversation with the Patient and, hopefully, Family. Both Patient and Clinician keep a copy of the order set. POLST instructs all providers regarding Patient preferences across care settings and/or in case of emergency. The forms and terminology of these order sets vary by state. Every Clinician should be aware of their state's requirements. The National POLST form and guide for use can be found in Appendix B.11.

While a Patient may have an AD without an agent, ADs encourage the designation of a Medical Durable Power of Attorney (MDPOA). The MDPOA is the legally designated decision-maker for the Patient when the Patient is unable to make their wishes known. Using the Patient's AD and their healthcare team as a guide, the MDPOA makes healthcare decisions based on what they understand of the specific situation, within the context of the Patient's values.

Sudden death disrupts the Healthcare Collaboration. Everyone's worse nightmare becomes real, including the Clinician's. In following the Buckman Protocol, establishing a safe space for delivering bad news is essential. The Family may be unable to absorb the reality. Reactions span the entire spectrum of human response, including emotional and physical behaviors. In sudden death, Family will need to hear of their loved one's demise multiple times and in many versions.

Futility

The American Medical Association (2007) has addressed the dire need for clearer communications and Advance Directives (AD) in its 2006 statement. Futility is defined as the process by which a Clinician may declare continued or proposed therapy to be futile (Fleming, 2005). Thus, continuation of care is unethical and may cause undue suffering and harm to the Patient and Family. In this statement, the AMA formally recognized the inescapable damage to all involved in futile Patient care. The 2016 AMA Code on Futility link can be found in Appendix B.12.

BOX 11.4 ANGIE

Long before the advent of Advance Directives, the ER received a nursing home patient. Angie was 94 years old, with a history of dementia and multiple admissions for urosepsis. As the EMT wheeled her into the medical bay, nursing reported her blood pressure was sinking rapidly. She was in septic shock. The resident, new to the unit, ordered IVs, antibiotics, and vasopressors for the central venous line he was about to place in her chest. The chief of service came up behind him, placing a hand on his shoulder. As the resident glanced back to his boss, the chief simply stated, "Don't just do something, stand there." The resident realized what the chief meant. Instead of a full code, the patient was given quiet comfort care until she died.

Relational Care is based on shared values, respect, and humanity. Recognizing futility prevented painful and pointless resuscitation.

Integration

Recent studies have shown that integration of care is expanding successfully outside the hospice, palliative care arenas. Having a difficult conversation is daunting. *Caring* for Patients requires more than delivering a pathology report or plan for therapy. Telling bad news involves the Personal and Relational Systems. As each individual receives the bad news, their reactions and growth into their new role must be reflected by the Healthcare Collaboration. Even when cure is not possible, healing can still occur.

Questions for Reflection

1   Have you or a family member ever received bad news? What was good about it? What was bad about it?
2   Have you ever had to deliver bad news as a provider? What was good about it? What bad about it?

References

American Medical Association. (2007). *Statement on end of life care.* AMA ethics resource center. Retrieved January 22, 2007, from www.ama-assn.org/ama/pub/category/7567.html

American Medical Association. (2016). *E-2.037 Medical futility in end-of-life care.* AMA code of ethics. Retrieved September 15, 2021, from www.ama-assn.org/ama/pub/category/8390.html

Borneman, T., Ferrell, B., & Puchalski, C. (2010). Evaluation of the FICA tool for spiritual assessment. *Journal of Pain and Symptom Management, 40*(2), 163–173. https://doi.org/10.1016/j.jpainsymman.2009.12.019

Buckman, R. (1992). *How to break bad news.* Johns Hopkins University Press.

Fleming, D. (2005). Futility: Revisiting a concept of shared moral judgement. *HEC Forum, 17*(4), 260–275. https://doi.org/10.1007/s10730-005-52253-z

Joint Commission. (2018). *Part 1. Body, mind, spirit.* The Source: For Joint Commission Compliance Strategies, *16*(1). Electronically retrieved from store.jcrinc.com/assets/1/14/ts_16_2018_01.

Luce, J., & Rubenfeld, G. (2002). Can health care costs be reduced by limiting intensive care at the end of life? *American Journal of Respirator Critical Care Medicine, 165,* 750–754. https://doi.org/10.1164/rccm.2109045

Motely, M. (2013). Advanced care planning. *Journal of American Academy of Physician Assistants, 20,* 6. https://doi.org/10.1097/01.jaa.0000430339.10272.9e

Siegel, B. (1998). *Peace, love, and healing.* Collins Publishers.

Sulmasy, D. (2006). Spiritual issues in the care of dying patients: . . . "it's okay between me and god". *Journal of American Medical Association, 296*(11), 1385–1392. https://doi.org/10.1001/jama.296.11.1385

12

BRIDGING THE GAP

Objectives

1   Recognize communication gaps
2   Understand presence and empathy
3   Learn and use the Four C's©
4   Understand the techniques of reframing, motivational interviewing, and the importance of empowerment

It is impossible not to communicate. Communication is basic interaction among people. The challenge of good communication involves concentration and paying attention. Miscommunication may be intentional or subconscious. Ineffective communication can result in dangerous, if not lethal, outcomes (Tiwary et al., 2019). This chapter focuses on problems caused by poor, incomplete, misguided, and insufficient communication.

Clinicians are taught specific communication tools during their formal training. Histories and Physicals, orders formats, consult notes, postoperative notes, discharge summaries, and SOAP notes (Subjective, Objective, Assessment, and Plan) are a fraction of written communication. Oral communication, especially when asking for input, can be misleading or unclear. Although formal communication skills are taught in medical education, communicating clearly with Patients is rarely, if ever, addressed (Tiwary et al., 2019).

Many factors influence poor communication such as hierarchical reporting structure, gender, education, cultural background, stress, fatigue, ethnic differences, and social structure (Shahid & Thomas, 2018). Originally developed to eliminate human error in communication during military operations, Situation, Background, Assessment, and Recommendation (SBAR) has been incorporated into medicine. Adapted in nursing communication with physicians, SBAR is now

DOI: 10.4324/9781003257219-16

TABLE 12.1 Situation, Background, Assessment, Recommendation (SBAR) Tool for Improved Communication Between Providers

Name	Definition	Components	Suggestions
Situation	What is going on with the patient	Your name, patient name, room number, reason for call	Have ALL data available including chart, medication, vital signs, recent labs, etc.
Background	Immediate and pertinent medical history pertaining to call	Medication list, IV fluids, vital signs, pertinent changes, clinical context	Specific data prompting call, exam findings, etc.
Assessment	What caller suspects or what they expect to occur as result of call	Suspected diagnosis, differential diagnoses	Suggestions of additional testing, studies, and/or therapies
Plan	Recommendations for additional therapies, testing	If appropriate, listing actions implemented or planned, including interventions	List diagnostic studies and interventions, when they should be completed and suggestions for additional therapies and studies

Source: Adapted from Studer Group (2007)

common in various specialties including anesthesia, pre-operative and postoperative medicine, obstetrics, emergency medicine, and acute care medicine (see Table 12.1).

When used in "handing off" a patient, SBAR has been shown to improve clinician-to-clinician communication. Awareness of the personal systems of other parties involved – Patient, Family, and Clinicians – improves efficiency and avoids conflict.

Multidisciplinary teams include members from diverse backgrounds and specialties. Today's common team members include lead physician, consultant services, PAs, NPs, and RNs. In addition, respiratory therapists, physical therapists, mental health therapists, case managers, social workers, chaplains, etc. play an integral role in cases. Insights from these specialists might not be obvious. However, their input is important to a broader perspective. Relational Care, as a systemic paradigm, values and utilizes the entire multidisciplinary team.

Relational Care recognizes gaps in communication and gives practitioners tools to manage them. This therapeutic model develops skills in giving bad news and working with different populations and cultures. In a medical crisis, it is impossible to think, much less communicate clearly, when processing life and death decisions. Even the most "centered" people are challenged in these circumstances.

Patients and Families process differently than Clinicians. As opposed to what they actually feel, many Patients and Families will respond to their interpretation of what the Clinician wants to hear. This results in miscommunication which may lead to suboptimal treatment decisions.

BOX 12.1   CHARLIE

Families can be left out of the process entirely or respond emotionally when faced with a crisis decision.

> *Fran, a Physician Assistant, was working in the ED when Charlie arrived. Awake and oriented, he reported having the flu the week before. Charlie thought he was improving, even his asthma was better. Suddenly, this morning, he began to feel short of breath. Despite using his rescue inhaler, Charlie was worsening, prompting his visit to the hospital. As the staff began Charlie's treatment and workup, he went into frank respiratory failure. Intubation was difficult. The Clinicians realized that his lack of response was not due to incorrect tube placement, but the lack of compliance in his lungs. Charlie was in status asthmaticus, a severe asthma attack.*
>
> *As the staff struggled to push air into Charlie's lungs, Fran's supervisory physician asked her to go talk to the Family regarding his sudden and life-threatening complication. Initially, only Charlie's sister was in the waiting room. She told Fran that Charlie felt so much better today that he decided to snort a line of cocaine. The drug, in addition to residual inflammation from the flu, triggered the asthma attack. As Fran quickly tried to describe Charlie's potentially fatal situation, his parents arrived. Devastated and hysterically crying, the mother began screaming. The sister became angry, asserting Charlie was talking when she brought him in.*
>
> *With the vital information regarding Charlie's cocaine use, Fran returned to the code. Despite the team's best efforts, his prognosis was poor. The physician in charge of the code asked Fran if the family understood what was happening and if they were "prepared." She replied, "I'm not going back out there, if that's what you mean! I've done the best I can with this family."*

Charlie's use of cocaine explained his acute presentation and his dismal prognosis. The family last saw him improving. Charlie's mild exacerbation of asthma appeared to them to be an easily controlled, routine ED visit. The family's anger was understandable. Their expectations were inconsistent with what they heard from Fran. The intensity of their reaction blocked any attempt at further communication.

Medical professionals are trained in delaying their emotional responses in crisis. Controlling their own emotions and their reactions to others leaves Clinicians both puzzled and stressed. This mix, powerful yet dysfunctional, leads to misunderstanding and malpractice suits.

Different mediating circumstances interfere with clear communication. It is important to be cognizant of Patient and Family expectations. For example, doctors and medical personnel are put on pedestals. Families expect that they should have all the answers regarding disease and treatment.

Additionally, most medical issues have more than one solution. Patients and Family become overwhelmed. They become incapable of choosing among multiple treatment options and their consequences. When the Clinician does not have a single, clear answer, expectations are dashed. Anger from the grief of bad news may devolve into threats of litigation.

Presence

"Staying in the moment" defines presence. It is the ability to eliminate distractions of personal Body, Mind, and Spirit to concentrate on the task at hand. Presence is listening with your eyes, your ears, and your heart. Conscious suspension of personal "stuff," when treating a Patient, is attention to the *Patient's* Body, Mind, and Spirit. There is no expectation or judgment. Being present is more than professional demeanor in the exam room. Clinical skills, senses, intuition, and *Spirit* are incorporated into connection with the Patient.

Both Venn diagrams (see Figures 2.2 and 2.3) reflect presence. The Personal and Relational Systems illustrate connections of Patient, Family, and Clinician. Appreciating the Personhood of each is therapeutic in itself.

The Healthcare Collaboration describes the Personal and Relational systems working together in the "sweet spots." Utilizing verbal and nonverbal communication creates relationships during interactions. The art of mirroring is a technique encouraging the Clinician to use the same body language as the Patient. Using the same gestures, expressions, vocal pitch, and tone reflects and strengthens rapport (Shellenbarger, 2016). A safe and intimate conversation develops an environment of trust. Having empathy is necessary for this process.

BOX 12.2   JACK

Jack was a successful PA with impressive credentials and reputation. His marriage, however, was in serious trouble. Walt was the Marriage and Family Therapist who recognized Jack and Kim needed to work on individual issues outside of conjoint sessions. During the customary individual therapeutic conversation, Walt suggested reviewing Jack's personal loss history might be helpful. Very reluctantly and with gentle support, Jack completed the task. At this point, Jack positioned himself as far away from Walt as physically possible. Walt enquired, "Have you ever cried for all of these losses?" Jack replied, "If I start, I'll never be able to stop."

> *As tears began to flow, Walt sat next to Jack and without touching him, he mirrored the grieving PA's body language. A trained therapist, Walt knew this was not the time for a hug. Presence, empathy, and mirroring were the prescriptions for the moment.*

Reframing uses alternative language to change the perspective of a situation, circumstance, or event. The classic example is the "glass half empty" versus "glass half full." By reframing, the Clinician facilitates a shift in understanding, establishing congruence.

Empathy is understanding another's feelings and emotions as if they were your own. Sympathy, which is feeling pity or sorrow for another's misfortunes, is nonproductive.

BOX 12.3   CRYSTAL

Dr. Bellow was a leading oncology surgeon. With a reputation for terrorizing students and residents, he was not known for his gentle nature. Crystal had been referred to him for her confirmed breast cancer. During her workup, a separate primary tumor was found in the contralateral breast. At the time, guidelines called for bilateral modified radical mastectomies. Crystal was distraught about the surgery. Her body image was important to her. Her impending disfigurement caused much of her distress.

The day after her surgery, Dr. Bellow and his full entourage rounded on all postoperative patients. As they entered her room, Crystal was quietly crying with her husband. Dr. Bellow asked if she was in pain. She shook her head no.

Dr. Bellow sat down on the edge of her bed and grasped both her hands in his. As she looked up into his eyes, he said, "You no longer have cancer in your body. THAT's what makes you beautiful."

Understanding Crystal's concerns of body image, Dr. Bellow was present to his Patient by showing empathy. He read her emotional pain and reframed Crystal's perspective in a positive light. Learning new insights beyond surgical skills, his team witnessed this moment of healing.

The Four C's©

Families and MDPOAs, in the agony of indecision, need the assurance and comfort of knowing the patient's values and wishes. Despite implementation of SPIKES and ADs (see Chapter 11), consensus breaks down in crisis. Having a "toolbox" of communication phrases brings clarity and understanding to each perspective. Known as "the Four C's$^{©}$" (Davenport & Schopp, 2014), simple use of words defuses and deescalates conflict. When used intentionally, CARE, CURIOUS, CONFUSED, and CONCERNED invite a nonconfrontational and nonjudgmental discussion. Promoting a safe forum for exchanging and questioning treatment options involves the entire Healthcare Collaboration. Valuing the contribution of all members allows opportunity to be "heard" in a time of chaos.

Expressing CARE facilitates attention and focus. The Clinician establishes his/her reason for being present – to support decision-makers. Affirming the Clinician is on "their side" removes barriers of a "we-them" agenda. "I CARE" expresses the Clinician's investment and sensitivity to Patient and Family. Difficult healthcare decisions must be reached with every member's input. Caring is a nonjudgmental stance that promotes productive dialogue.

Being CURIOUS seeks understanding of an expressed rationale. The Patient is the expert in what is happening to their Body. With CURIOUS questions, the Clinician is deferring to the Patient. Family, friends, and caregivers can only reflect what THEY see and experience. Curiosity (with attention to Body, Mind, and Spirit) generates needed information in a gentle, nonthreatening manner.

When we are CONFUSED, we simply do not understand. As the Clinician expresses confusion, permission for clarification is encouraged. The resulting explanation expands options which eventually leads to negotiation. Instead of a definitive statement, being CONFUSED leads to individualized input and subtle changes. Patient, family members, and/or other Clinicians are asked to explain their rationale. As the plan develops, everyone is "on the same page." Defending a position is no longer necessary. Trust and consensus build as the solution becomes the focus.

BOX 12.4 MRS. CARTER

Choosing words carefully shifts the environment and empowers input from Patient, Family, and Clinician

Mrs. Carter was a 75-year-old cancer patient. Her tumor was large, requiring extensive surgery. Therefore, she was referred to a major teaching hospital. As the surgeon, Dr. Henry, described the procedure and recovery process, Mrs. Carter brought up other tests and studies. Sensing her hesitancy, Dr. Henry stated, "I'm confused, I thought you wanted to proceed with surgery right away." His "confusion" gave her permission to respond. Mrs. Carter explained her recovery would mean she would miss her granddaughter's graduation followed by a family reunion that weekend. Once

> *Dr. Henry was aware of the celebration, a delay in the surgery was quickly negotiated.*

Dr. Henry understood his Patient recognized his authority. Being CONFUSED increased Mrs. Carter's comfort level and empowered her to express her concerns. Without Dr. Henry's invitation to share, Mrs. Carter would have missed a critical milestone in her Family story.

CONCERN is reflected as a component of caring *and* the medical expertise of the Clinician. It implies there is no complete agreement or consensus. Being CONCERNED suggests better options exist. It allows for explanation of the rationale resulting from disparity within the Healthcare Collaboration. Input from patient, family members, specialists, and others *and* the time for consultation may be necessary to satisfy CONCERN.

CONSENSUS is the goal of using the Four C's©. Reaching CONSENSUS is the assurance that all parties understand and respect the others' perspectives. It is autonomous decision-making, true Informed Consent. The Healthcare Collaboration is the agreement of the Personal and Relational Systems – when both "sweet spots" of the Venn diagrams align. CONSENSUS is the culmination of all input from Patient, Family, and Clinician. It results in a treatment plan customized to the care of the Patient's Body, Mind, and Spirit. Using the Four C's, the Healthcare Collaboration unites in CONSENSUS.

Motivational Interviewing

Medical interviewing is an art and skill simultaneously. A systems perspective empowers the Clinician to choose to stray from the "protocol pathway" by including Motivational Interviewing (MI). MI is a communication tool to attain a goal, using language of *change*. It is a collaborative process involving the Patient and Clinician. Listening empathetically, without interruption, a Clinician sees, hears, and feels how they can encourage a positive outcome.

BOX 12.5 GEORGE

Emphasizing the impact of deleterious behavior of a Patient's lifestyle, MI supports and guides the Patient to choose a healthy balance. Compliance is *enabled* because the Patient makes the decision.

> *George was a 62-year-old truck driver. He arrived at the Veteran's Administration Hospital with a classic case of peripheral vascular disease resulting*

in a mummified second toe. His physical exam revealed absent pulses in the Dorsalis pedis and Posterior tibialis arteries. Standard treatment, for this presentation, was aorto-bifemoral grafting with a partial amputation of his toe. George refused, stating he was scared of the surgery. The surgeon asked if he was willing to try an alternative treatment.

Hearing that his two packs a day habit was the main contributor to his disease state, George declared he had just smoked his last cigarette. He agreed to think about surgery, begin a walking regimen, and return in 6 weeks for a follow-up appointment.

George's follow-up exam revealed the distal portion of his toe had fallen off, leaving a clean, well-healed surface that was not causing him symptoms. His pulses had improved to a +1 Dorsalis pedis and +2 Posterior tibialis. George's exercise tolerance had increased. Surgery was no longer indicated. George was empowered to continue his healthier lifestyle.

Empowerment

The savvy, mature diagnostician teases out the correct diagnosis after others fail. Sometimes, their abilities appear almost magical because they ask the same questions. The interview protocol is standardized. The difference is not in the method of data gathering but in the openness of the Clinician.

Empowering the Patient, the Personhood of the Clinician listens *and* responds to the Personhood of the Patient. This is a subtle but powerful acknowledgment that the Patient is the expert of his/her Body.

BOX 12.6 ROXY

Empowerment is not only for those who need care but also for caregivers.

Roxy was a PA with 18 years of experience in Family Practice Medicine. Her parents lived 15 minutes away, creating an ideal work/life balance. Her two children, aged 6 and 4, were still asleep early one morning when a call from her mother came. Roxy's father was feeling bad, having shortness of breath and mild chest pain. She urged her mother to call 911, woke her husband, and slipped on some clothes.

By the time Roxy arrived at her parent's house, Emergency Medical Services (EMS) was on site. As she entered her parent's bedroom, Roxy saw them performing CPR. With difficulty, they stabilized her father for transfer.

In ICU, Roxy's grave assessment was confirmed. The intensivist asked about her father's end-of-life preferences. Distraught, Roxy's mother turned to her for an answer.

> *Roxy asked for some time to think. The physician agreed, saying he would be in the unit for the rest of his shift, available as needed. As he left the room, he leaned over to Roxy and quietly stated, "You don't need to be a PA right now. You need to be a daughter."*

Relational Care is a visually simple concept. It empowers each member of the Healthcare Collaboration (Patient, Family, and Clinician) to do whatever they need to do. For example, Patients ask questions to clarify their confusion and worry. "How long will I be out of work?" "When will I be able to leave the hospital?"

The Family has its own set of questions regarding the disease impacting their loved one and Family. "Will she be okay?" "Does he need to have someone with him all the time?" "How can we pay the medical bills?" "Will I/we be okay?"

The Clinician questions "Have we considered all available treatment options?" "Do I have all of the psychosocial information I need?" "Do I understand what the Patient wants?"

These questions have everything to do with Personhood. With Relational Care, every encounter becomes more than a History of Present Illness, Review of Systems, and paternalistic Assessment and Plan. Informed Consent is not merely a sheet of paper with obligatory signatures. Rather, all parties together develop the individualized treatment plan, promoting understanding, compliance, and satisfaction. The Clinician empowers the Patient and Family as advocates. Every element is respected and valued.

Discerning what a loved one would want is never easy. An Advance Directive (AD) and a designated Medical Durable Power of Attorney (MDPOA) protect wishes. This is a difficult and necessary conversation (Davenport & Schopp, 2011). Many families expect Clinicians to initiate this conversation (Balaban, 2000).

Revisiting and updating Patient wishes and expectations need to occur on a regular basis. As the experts in the Patient's clinical course and prognosis, it is incumbent upon Clinicians to keep the Healthcare Collaboration updated. This gives the MDPOA a timeline along with the prognosis. The timeline need not be precise but helps prepare the MDPOA and the Family.

Attorneys, especially those trained in elder care law, can assist in this process. Legal and medical communities have forms for ADs and MDPOA designation. Seniors' mentation can vacillate according to time of day, medication, and overall health. Assessing a patient's "best time" assures competency regarding preferences for personal and medical care. Advocacy is the process of expressing and appreciating the values and ethics of self and others (Sulmasy, 2006). It is the duty of each member of the Healthcare Collaboration to advocate for each other and themselves. The MDPOA is the designated Patient advocate. They rely on input from Clinicians and Family to act upon Advance Directives. Advocacy tends to promote itself. As the Healthcare Collaboration (see Figures 2.2 and 2.3) advocates and promotes its members, the members are empowered to help others. As consensus builds, care for the Patient and each other evolves.

Questions for Reflection

1   Review the case study in Textbox 12.1. How would you use the Four C's in communicating with the Family?
2   How do you resolve conflict? With your family, friends, and peers?

References

Balaban, R. (2000). A physician's guide to talking about end-of-life care. *Journal of Internal Medicine, 15*(3), 195–200. https://doi.org/10.1046/j.1525-1497.2000.07228.x

Davenport, L., & Schopp, G. (2011). Breaking bad news: Communication skills for difficult conversations. *Journal for the American Academy of Physician Assistant, 24*(2), 46–50. https://doi.org/10.1097/01720610-201102000-00008

Davenport, L., & Schopp, G. (2014). When communication fails: Resolving end of life impasses. *Journal for the American Academy of Physician Assistant, 27*(6), 28–31. https://doi.org/10/1097/01.JAA.0000444733.31916.2b

Shahid, S., & Thomas, S. (2018). Situation, background, assessment, recommendation (SBAR) communication tool for handoff in health care- A narrative review. *Safety in Health, 4*(7). https://doi.org/10.1186/s40886-018-0073-1

Shellenbarger, S. (2016, September 20). Use mirroring to connect with others. *The Wall Street Journal 3. Retrieved from www.wsj.com*

Studer Group. (2007). *Patient safety toolkit- Practical tactics that improve both patient safety and patient perceptions of care.* Studer Group.

Sulmasy, D. (2006). Spiritual issues in the care of dying patients: . . . "it's okay between me and god". *Journal of American Medical Association, 296*(11), 1385–1392. https://doi.org/10.1001/jama.296.11.1385

Tiwary, A., Rimal, A., Paudyal, B., Sigdel, K., & Basnyat, B. (2019). Poor communication by heath care professionals may lead to life-threatening complications: Examples from two case reports. *Wellcome Open Research, 4*(2). https://doi.org/10.12688/welcomeopenres.15042.1

13

TAKING CARE OF THE CAREGIVER

Objectives

1   Understand the importance of self-care
2   Develop self-care strategies

Introduction

Caregiving is not a job or a career. It is a calling that requires openness to another in their suffering. There are professional and nonprofessional caregivers. The amount of caregiving directly correlates with increased levels of stress (Pearlin et al., 1990). When the intensity of caregiving escalates, so does the danger of compassion fatigue and burnout.

Self-care management maintains caregiver health. Recognition that there is a problem and knowing steps to prevent damage is necessary for Patient, Family, and Clinician, aka "caregivers." Strategies and resources need to be in place BEFORE they are required.

Self-care is care of the Body, Mind, and Spirit. Caregivers, particularly Clinicians, have been trained and take pride in their ability to deny care of self in service. However, without conscious, disciplined care, they will eventually burnout.

Imagine the metaphor of a caregiver as a pitcher of water. A big pitcher of ice-cold water on a hot day is not only desirable, it is necessary. Filling cups with water for everyone who is thirsty brings comfort and relief from the heat. Like the pitcher of water, caregivers give of themselves, filling empty cups. If the water pitcher is not refilled on a regular basis, everyone thirsts. Caregivers require replenishment. The water pitcher empties faster with the following:

A.   Countertransference impacts healthcare encounters. Cautionary Issues, Chapter 9, describes its influence on Patient, Family, and Clinician relationships. Countertransference cannot be ignored. Awareness of it reduces negative experiences.

DOI: 10.4324/9781003257219-17

B. Maintaining clear boundaries is a challenge. Boundaries are the distinction of being oneself by separation from thoughts, feelings, behaviors, and actions of another. Good boundaries are protective and permeable. They allow connection with Patients and Family without jeopardizing the Clinician.

BOX 13.1   NICK

Hospitalized that evening for a relatively simple exacerbation of his COPD, Nick was driving the staff to distraction. He constantly requested to have his providers paged. During rounds the following day, the Clinician brought up Nick's frequent calls. Recognizing that his behavior was due to shortness of breath and anxiety, the Clinician assured Nick he was being closely monitored. He offered to round on him twice a day. With increased monitoring, Nick's anxiety diminished, resulting in a marked improvement in his symptoms and reduced calls for care.

Clear boundary setting benefited both Patient and Clinician. Communication reduced the Patient's anxiety and his demands on the Clinician's time.

Establishing boundaries is a necessary life skill. They are used in all social settings including personal, family, peer, and professional interactions.

C. Balance is intrinsic to well-being. It is a process of conscious and regular assessment, giving attention to needs of the Body, Mind, and Spirit, as they develop. For example, eating for nutrition and to satiate hunger maintains physical health. Eating out of boredom or as a coping mechanism is physically and psychologically unhealthy. A balanced life facilitates successful adaptation to life changes.

D. Sometimes Clinicians resort to black humor to cope with the stress. What may seem to be inappropriate is, in fact, a commentary on the high stakes of the clinical situation. Black humor, also known as gallows humor, breaks tension and facilitates "reboot" of the thought process. It is a balancing strategy to support clinical effectiveness.

BOX 13.2   BLACK HUMOR TO COPE WITH STRESS

The surgical team spent over an hour isolating the large mass in the patient's neck. It was exhausting, tedious work. The six cm mass was finally freed and lifted out. The surgeon marked the boundaries, handed it back to the tech, and ordered, "Spank it, give it a name, and take the APGAR."

> The entire team was tired and tense. The tumor's size and malignancy potential added to the stress. The relief of excising the mass was overshadowed by the awareness of the work still ahead. Black humor acknowledged the accomplishment while preparing the team. It is often used in extreme, stressful environments.

Humor provides a mental and emotional break. Laughter is a form of communication that relieves stress and establishes camaraderie. Humor does not decrease stress. Rather, it *increases* the ability to cope (Thorson & Powell, 2006).

Self-Care Strategies

The effectiveness of the Healthcare Collaboration relies on optimum functioning. Relational Care focuses attention on care of Body, Mind, and Spirit. Self-care strategies restore balance to the system and support Personhood. Successful strategies are unique and personal. What works for the individual is a lifelong learning process. William Worden (2002) provides a self-care checklist for each practitioner summarized in Table 13.1.

Workplace interventions and trainings are effective at recognizing and controlling the symptoms of Compassion Fatigue and Burnout Syndrome. Mindfulness training programs improve self-compassion and reduce emotional exhaustion in healthcare providers (Gozalo et al., 2019). Benefits include reductions in blood pressure, depression, and anxiety (Goldstein et al., 2012).

Mindfulness practice is a meditative process that uses the Mind and Body to concentrate and subsequently relax. Simple acts of purposeful, slow deep breathing regenerates Body, Mind, and Spirit. Mindfulness is the root of consciousness, attention, and awareness.

The internet provides many resources on the practice of mindfulness. A basic exercise starts by finding a comfortable, quiet, place to sit. Breathe deeply and slowly to a count of three, in through the nose and expanding the diaphragm. Blow out through the mouth to another slow count of three. Keep a slow and steady tempo while concentrating on breathing. As attention wanders, gently refocus on

TABLE 13.1 Personal Care Checklist: Originally Developed by Dr. Kubler-Ross and Adapted by Dr. William Worden (2002)

Know your limits
Practice active grieving
Practice healthy living
Recognize personal mortality
Accept the profession as a calling

the rising and falling of the chest. Develop self-compassion by not judging the exercise. Set a timer for five minutes to avoid "watching the clock."

Deep breathing along with clenching and relaxing muscles is another opportunity for stress reduction and relaxation promotion. Count and regulate breathing, tighten muscle groups starting with the toes and working up to the forehead. Try to isolate each group. For example, tighten toes . . . two . . . three . . . relax . . . two . . . three. Do this twice before moving up to ankles. Concentrate on maintaining a slow, steady pace. Attention to detail provides greater relaxation and stress relief. This exercise is particularly helpful in bed when preparing to sleep.

Guided imagery expands on the breathing exercise by focusing on a choice of person, place, and circumstance. For example, a trained facilitator guides visualization to a safe and relaxing place. Using a thoughtful and conscious process, awareness of sounds, colors, smells, etc., is accessed and developed. The result of the experience is discussed with the facilitator, allowing access to the visualization at any time.

Performing a simple act using mindfulness techniques is another way to reduce stress. Merely washing hands, while concentrating on both breathing and the task, will regulate breathing, lower blood pressure, and clear thinking.

During the COVID pandemic, the Society of Critical Care Medicine recognized the increased stress on Clinicians. It introduced the practice of wellness in its blog (2020). In co-operation with the American Psychiatry Association, Clinicians were encouraged to use a simple grounding exercise. "Grounding" emphasizes the concentration on the five senses in the present moment. In a quiet moment, notice the following:

- Five things you can see
- Four things you can feel or touch
- Three things you can hear
- Two things you can smell
- One thing you can taste

Additional strategies include consciously observing nature for a specific period of time. Maintaining social connections with friends and co-workers, in different environments, promotes emotional and mental health. Self-rewards for completion of tasks, like a five-minute break outside, refresh perspective and reset the mind for what is next.

Leaving the work role at work is difficult. Allow five minutes to reset before getting in the car. Use drive time to listen to favorite music. The car becomes a safe space in transitioning roles from Clinician to Family member.

A healthy Body involves establishing and maintaining physical health. The mantra of eating properly, exercising regularly, and developing good sleep habits are all part of the formula. The discipline required to follow the formula is easily derailed by work, family, and community needs.

A healthy Mind requires both stimulation and rest. Reading a "fun" book, playing a game, working a puzzle, or taking a walk are examples of diversionary rest. Hobbies are low stakes distractions that provide problem-solving satisfaction and accomplishment. Knowing one's limits, through reflective writing, journaling, or meditation, allows the Mind to process and reorder priorities.

A healthy Spirit develops through self-reflection. Spiritual health habits include opening the mind through journaling, meditating, inspirational reading, and appreciating nature. Prayer, in whatever form, connects us to something spiritually outside of ourselves. Religion is but one road to the practice of spirituality.

"Technology abstinence" enables the Body, Mind, and Spirit to explore rest. Devices and technology are effusive and pervasive distractions. The bombardment of news bites, Tweets, texts, alerts, etc. is contrary to self-care. By demanding attention, devices have an addictive quality that prevents healthy renewal. The pressure of being connected digitally interferes with intra- and interpersonal depth.

Vacation may be defined as "recovery from work" (Bloom et al., 2012, p. 306). A lack of vacations has been linked to increased morbidity and mortality (Gump & Matthews, 2000). A change of scene, as in a vacation or conference, revives Personhood. New perspectives and opportunities enrich and feed our creativity and passion. For full benefits on health and well-being, "staycations" require experiences outside the normal routine. Any successful strategy includes new stimulation with sufficient time for rest and reflection (Sonnentag & Fritz, 2007).

Part of self-care is grieving loss. Recognizing that healthcare involves loss, a Clinician must address it. The utilization of a personal loss history (see Appendix B.3) is a tool to enable understanding of the process. It does not eliminate the need for grieving.

Supervision is a formal or informal conversation discussing a particular concern or question. Historically, supervision is perceived as weakness. Reaching out on a regular basis to talk and process is not only healthy, it also maintains professional effectiveness. Meeting with a higher level practitioner is an opportunity for growth.

BOX 13.3   PEER SUPERVISION

Another professional, unrelated to the problem, can give objective perspective.

Two mental health counselors and a Physician Assistant were having a casual conversation. The counselors were describing the distress of a sexually abused patient who did not like to be touched. The patient was unable to tolerate vital signs during a simple office visit. As the PA listened to her colleagues, she asked, "Why not teach the patient to take her own vitals?" Not only did this solution prevent the patient from the distress of being touched it, also empowered her with control of her body.

> Peer supervision takes place when a problem is brought before co-workers of the same level of expertise. The old adage of "two heads are better than one" was proven true. Casual conversation resulted in a creative solution through peer supervision.

Relying on and expanding the multidisciplinary team provides informal supervision with difficult cases.

As Clinicians, demands are many. There is never enough time. Professional caregivers are expected to respond immediately and competently. These stressors increase the likelihood of ignoring self-care. Compassion fatigue and burnout result from inattention to changes in attitude in Body, Mind, and Spirit. Maintaining boundaries and balance promote a positive work ethic and professional collaboration.

Informal caregivers are less likely to recognize compassion fatigue or burnout. Referral to appropriate providers maintains the health of informal and formal caregivers. Relational Care appreciates each individual's Personhood. Collaboration among Body, Mind, and Spirit of every member provides a working framework for support, perspective, and validation. Through open communication, Relational Care manages stress.

Self-Care Is Not an Option.

Questions for Reflection

1   Think about the last time you laughed at black humor. What changed?
2   If you do not take care of yourself, you will not be able to care for others. How are you taking care of yourself right now?
3   When was the last time you went on a technology vacation?

References

Bloom, J., Guerts, S., & Kompier, M. (2012). Effects of short vacations, vacation activities, and experiences on employee health and well-being. *Stress and Health, 28,* 306–318. https://doi.org/10.1002/smi.1434

Goldstein, C., Josephson, R., Xie, S., & Hughes, J. (2012). Current perspectives on the use of meditation to reduce blood pressure. *International Journal of Hypertension,* 578397. https://doi.org/10.1155/2012/578397

Gozalo, R., Tarres, J., Ayora, A., & Herrero, M. (2019). Application of a mindfulness program among healthcare professionals in an intensive care unit: Effect on burnout empathy and self-compassion. *Medicina Intensive, 43*(4), 207–216. https://doi.org/10.1016/j.medine.2019.03.006

Gump, B., & Matthews, K. (2000). Are vacations good for your health? The 9 – year mortality experience after the multiple risk factor intervention trial. *Psychosomatic Medicine, 62,* 608–612. https://doi.org/10/1097/00006842-200009000-00003

Pearlin, L., Mullan, J., Semple, S., & Skaff, M. (1990). Caregiving and the stress process: An overview of the concepts and their measures. *The Gerontologist, 30*(5), 583–594. https://doi.org/10.1093geront/30.5.583

Society of Critical Care Medicine. (2020, July). How to maintain wellness. *Society of Critical Care Medicine.* www.scc.org/Blog/July-2020/How-to-Maintain-Wellness-the-COVID-19-Pandemic

Sonnentag, S., & and Fritz, C. (2007). The recovery experience questionnaire: Development and validation of a measure for assessing recuperation and unwinding from work. *Journal of Occupational Health Psychology, 12,* 204–221. https://doi.org/10.1037/1076-8998.12.3.204

Thorson, J., & Powell, F. C. (2006). Development and validation of a multidimensional sense of humor scale. *Journal of Clinical Psychology, 19,* 13–23. https://doi.org/10/10002/1097-4679(199301)49:1 < 13::AID-JCLP2270490103 > 3.0.CO;2-S

Worden, W. (2002). *Grief counseling and grief therapy.* Springer Publishing.

APPENDIX A

Case Studies for Role Play

General Instructions: These role plays were developed to teach students how to tell "bad news." The SPIKE protocol (Chapter 11) is appropriate for other difficult encounters. The Four C's (Chapter 12) manage confrontation in clinical, professional, peer-to-peer, and personal situations. The goal of these tools is to improve communication and understanding, resulting in consensus.

The scenarios are best utilized starting with Role Play 1 for students without any coaching. The initial role play should not last more than five minutes. Subsequent role plays may run longer with interruptions for coaching. The entire class is presented with the Setup. Each actor receives a card describing their role.

Following the role play, each actor is asked to describe their experience. The rest of the class is invited to contribute their observations and personal experiences. No one is required to share. The instructor is responsible for creating a safe environment enabling self-disclosure.

After Role Play 1, class is taught the SPIKES protocol and the Four C's. The role play is repeated and modified using the new information. After each role play, the class, as a group or divided into small groups, discusses the following general questions.

1   How did you feel as you observed the role play?
2   To the actors, how did you feel about your role?
3   What did you notice?
4   What was most difficult? What was most helpful?
5   What did you need that was not available?
6   What have you learned?
7   Have you had a similar personal experience?
8   Could this scenario have been managed better? Why?

Another group of student actors is given a different scenario to role play with their newly acquired skills. Each student actor should receive a card with the scenario basics listed as well as their specific role. Coaching should be minimal, but if the student is obviously stuck, guidance should be available. Reading the text beforehand is helpful for students, but not necessary. Reviewing the questions after each role play clarifies and reinforces the lesson.

Role Play 1: Elder Care

Setup: The patient is a 93-year-old female who has been in long-term nursing home care with dementia, diabetes, hypertension, peripheral neuropathy, and vascular dementia/pin strokes. She has had three hospitalizations in the past year for urosepsis and failure to thrive. While the infections are easily controlled with appropriate therapy, she is experiencing a steady decline in her overall baseline and her Activities of Daily Living. She returns to the Emergency Department again with high fever, delirium, and urosepsis.

PA: You are a hospitalist in the local facility with a new patient who came in last night. Patient is a 93-year-old female with her fourth episode of urosepsis in the past year. She is currently running a fever of 102.8 orally and labs reveal poorly controlled DMT2, leukocytosis, and urinalysis with gross bacteria and WBCs. She has no Advance Directives, and her family is gathering in the patient's room per her MDPOA request.

Daughter A: You are the daughter with MDPOA, the only family left in town to help Mom during her decline. You've seen Mom become progressively more miserable and demented through this past year. She gets markedly worse each time she requires hospital care. She doesn't seem to improve much when she finally gets home. In fact, the only time she brightens up is when she sees your daughter. Many times, she calls your daughter by your name, but you think that's because you looked so similar when you were her age. You want Mom back in the nursing home. You're in danger of losing your job because you've missed so much work while she's hospitalized. You don't see an end to this, you're exhausted, scared of making a bad decision, angry that it's all on you.

Patient: You are a grandmother with dementia. Your confusion increases the sicker you become. You love your children and sometimes forget their names. Calling everyone "honey" seems to be easier than trying to remember. You do know the little girl who eats ice cream with you is makes you feel good. She looks like, no, she IS your oldest daughter. You tend to also mistake your other children for long-dead relatives. You don't feel bad, but you haven't felt good in a long time.

Grandchild, A$_1$: You are 10 years old and you are back in this scary place because of something bad with your Grannie. You love visiting Grannie in the nursing home. There, you are instantly "her baby" and get to sit in her lap eating ice cream. Your attention getting behavior usually gets you what you want. Mom is becoming increasingly distant to you every time Grannie is in the hospital.

Eldest Son A: You are the male, the patriarch of the family since Dad died 6 years ago. You are the breadwinner for your own family, the successful one. You had to fly in last night. A new contract is due. You're getting phone calls about the fine details. You are the Man in Charge. You feel like you should take charge of this situation like you would at your job. But this is confusing and uncomfortable. You want Mom healthy and well. You KNOW more can be done if you can only figure out how to get past this stupid PA and talk to the "real doctor."

Daughter B: You live out of state and have flown in for this emergency conference about Mom. You are irritated about your sister's (Daughter A) inability to keep things under control. You chose to be out of the loop, making you feel guilty. Seeing Mom today escalates your guilt- you want EVERYTHING done. You ask questions, but you are not interested in answers that do not allay your fears. You just want Mom taken care of so you can go home.

Instructor Notes: This case is an introduction to role play. The instructor should encourage volunteers to participate freely in their roles. Although each role is well described, some students will need encouragement and suggestions on assuming their character.

No props are necessary, but physical setup is required. The patient, PA, the MDPOA (daughter A), and granddaughter (A_1) should be together initially. The other actors join later, as prompted by the instructor. A_1, the 10-year-old granddaughter, needs to act like a brat, for example. The PA should be in a hurry, a little frustrated that the family cannot see the obvious trajectory of the patient's course. Choosing a female PA illustrates gender issues with the "take charge" son.

Traditionally, this case study introduces the lecture on how to tell "bad news." After describing SPIKES and the Four C's©, the case study can be repeated. Coaching from instructor and feedback from the class should be encouraged.

Role Play 2: Terminal Care

Setup: The Patient is a 45-year-old female with a 4-year history of ovarian cancer. Classed as Stage III on diagnosis, the cancer has steadily progressed. Now the Patient is failing all therapies. She has undergone repeated abdominal paracentesis for recurrent malignant ascites. Chemotherapy and cachexia have turned her into a walking ghost. She has marginal quality of life but has fought hard with the loving support of her family. She is so tired.

PA: You are seeing the patient for evaluation before her paracentesis and chemotherapy. She is experiencing a slow but marked decline, accelerating in the past several months. You've been involved with her fight from Day 1 of the diagnosis. You know the family and how they support and love her. You see an ill and exhausted patient before you.

Patient: You are a 45-year-old terminal ovarian cancer patient. Despite your determination to stay alive and keep your family going, you know you are dying. You are miserable. The chemotherapy has you sick, not just the day after, but constantly. Your oncologist has a new therapy that is investigational but appears to have "great promise." You just want to go home. You want to spend the time you have left with your family.

MD: You breeze into the room with your PA to describe the newest therapy you just ordered for your patient. "Begood" is a promising new drug with supposedly fewer side effects and "maybe" a better 5-year survival rate. Nothing else is working in this case, so why not? You rattle off a few numbers on "5-year survival, tumor load regression, and side effects" (Actor note: Make them up, no one is listening, much less remembering the specifics at this point) and leave the room before the hard questions start. You have 20 more patients to see this morning.

Husband: You've watched your beloved wife soldier through countless procedures, chemos, pokes, and prods. You fear the future, you're angry at your inability to make a difference in her care or comfort. You're grieving as you watch her waste away into a ghost of the person she was. You are trying to hold the family together and you feel like you're failing. "Begood" could be the life preserver you've all been looking for. You are scared and hopeful at the same time.

Daughter: You are a 21-year-old college student. Mom and Dad urged you to go to your dream college, 4 hours away. You're having a blast and doing well in your major. You're back early for the weekend to visit and to give Dad a break. Your bond with Mom has always been special – shopping, cooking, chatting . . . She seems to be withdrawn lately, less likely to talk and smile even when reliving fond memories. It's harder to "get her back" every time you visit.

Son: You are 18 years old, in your last year of high school. Because of Mom's condition, your social life has been reduced to visiting hospital rooms and buying flowers for her. You're struggling in school because you don't know where you're supposed to be, much less what you're supposed to be doing. Dates are impossibly awkward now; you've forgotten how to laugh or have fun. You barely understand your Mom's diagnosis and you certainly don't want to talk about it with any of your peers. Your only release is football when you get to hit something. You barely have time for that anymore, even though Coach has been kind about the missed practices and games. You're trying to keep Dad's spirits up, you're not sure how to help him without making the both of you too uncomfortable. Mom is so fragile now. You feel awkward around her but are desperate for her touch because you love her.

Instructor Notes: The MD should leave after introducing the new chemotherapy. The PA remains to respond to questions and concerns.

This case illustrates the need for one-on-one conversations. Initially, seeing the Patient alone empowers his/her to discuss preferences. Remind students they are not responsible for alleviating mental or spiritual distress. Recommendations for spiritual and mental health specialists, hospice and palliative care, and support groups are appropriate. This is an excellent opportunity to address experiencing grief and loss as a caregiver (Chapters 8 and 13).

The Clinician learns how to advocate for their Patient by being present and listening to them without other Family members (Chapter 11). Being present is not only listening to what another is saying but it also includes observing body language, mirroring, and being comfortable with silences. Many Patients find it easier to say "yes" to continued treatment than trying to explain why they really want to say "no more." The Clinician, as advocate, may have to become the Patient's voice.

Role Play 3: Desperate Newlyweds

Setup: The Patient is a 65-year-old male with a long history of COPD and asthma. He was widowed over 20 years ago and he raised his two children alone after his wife's death. After a recent move, the patient met a divorced mother of three adult children. It was love at first sight. Their courtship was careful and slow. They married 6 months ago.

For the past 4 weeks, the patient noticed increasing right shoulder pain. The chest films were negative; however, the CT was ominous. A mass in the apex of the lung was subsequently confirmed as a Pancoast tumor. Fortunate to be near a major medical center, the patient entered aggressive therapy.

The patient underwent the full excision of the mass with an upper lobectomy and soft tissue extirpation. Prognosis was good. However, he suffered multiple recurrent pleural effusions that further compromised his already poor lung function. He required multiple thoracentesis procedures and suffered several bouts of pneumonia.

After a month in the hospital and rehab, the patient was able to go home. Less than 24 hours later, he returned to the hospital with a femoral artery embolus. During the embolectomy, a clot mobilized to the patient's carotid artery, resulting in a hemispheric stroke. He also developed dry gangrene of the great toe on the ipsilateral side. In the subsequent months, the patient suffered recurrent pleural effusions (reactive), pneumonias, progressive gangrene of the foot, and minimal improvement from the cerebral vascular accident. He underwent numerous codes secondary to sepsis, chronic and acute kidney failure, and respiratory failure.

The patient's new wife lived by his side, going home only to get fresh clothing. She was active in his therapy sessions and care. His wife described to the staff their continued "good life" as soon as he fully recovered.

Patient: A devote Catholic, you dearly love your new wife. She brought life back into your world and your kids adore her. Your Baptist wife is clearly devoted to you and strong in her faith. She prays daily with you and assures you things will improve.

You are in pain and breathing is a constant struggle. On the ventilator, you communicate with your eyes. You want to protect your wife. As a tough Vietnam vet, your helplessness and failure to improve are maddening.

Wife: After a horrible divorce, you've met the "man of your dreams." Your favorite name for your husband is "my Prince." Just like in the movies, you believe in your love for each other. Your prayers will result in a miracle, if you believe hard enough. Your husband needs to fight, to hang on until it comes. You will not discuss hospice care or End of Life. God will provide.

PA: As with so many other patients, you know where this ICU patient is headed. The only question in your mind is how long will it take for him to die. The patient has already survived four full codes and multiple procedures. Despite removal of the tumor, he still has cancer. His wife's devotion to his care and recovery is admirable. She is unrealistic in her expectations of his recovery. She frequently asks when he will be discharged home.

Earlier, you broached the topic of a DNR but was strongly rejected. With the patient's accelerating decline, you need to address Advance Directives again.

Instructor Notes: This role play demonstrates the importance of the SPIKES protocol (Chapter 11) when End-of-Life discussions are necessary. Each disease course change requires a review of Patient understanding and Advance Directives.

This case demonstrates miscommunication when each party in the Healthcare Collaboration is in a different place. No matter how the PA approaches the topic, the wife will deny her husband's eventual demise. Clinicians cannot "fix" this dynamic. They are responsible for communicating the status of the Patient and what the changes in status mean. Religious beliefs may contribute to how bad news is received.

A sample dialogue between the PA and the wife, outside of the patient's room can be given to students.

PA: Is this a good time to talk?

Wife: Yes, don't you think he's doing better? He had a good night.

PA: How do you think he's been doing this past week?

Wife: Well, this last infection was bad. When will he get off the ventilator?

PA: How much do you want to know about what happened last week?

Wife: He's getting better, right?

PA: He is improving for now. However, every time he has one of these incidents, he doesn't recover as fully as we would like. In other words, he is declining, overall.

Wife: Don't you say that in front of my husband! He IS getting better!

PA: I can see how much you care about each other. I care for both of you also. I'm trying to understand what your expectations are. I'm curious, what are YOUR questions about your husband's status?

Wife: It just seems like every time he starts to get better, he has another big setback. I just want to know when he can go home.

PA: Right now, he is unable to breathe without the ventilator. He can only stay off the machine for a few days. Each setback makes it less likely he will be able to breathe on his own.

Wife: Are you trying to tell me this is the way it's going to be . . . Forever?!

PA: I'm concerned. This is not what anyone wants to hear. Your husband is declining. We need to make some tough decisions. I would like to write an order for a hospice consultation. They can come to visit you and offer treatment options and services.

This case presents an opportunity for discussing futility and ethics consults.

Role Play 4: Drugged Heart

Setup: A 23-year-old crack and meth addict is admitted for the fourth time with congestive heart failure. His heart is huge, with an ejection fraction of less than 12%. He is otherwise healthy. He is not a candidate for a transplant because of his indigent status and positive drug screens.

Patient: You are only 23 years old and have been doing drugs since you were 15. You didn't start having trouble with shortness of breath and difficulty with exercise until about a year ago. You suspect you aren't getting help because you're black and that makes you angry. You are emotionally immature and unstable, becoming increasingly hostile and argumentative as the interview progresses. You believe they are using your drug use – just a few touches to keep withdrawal away – as an excuse to keep another black man down and out.

Mother: Despite your best efforts as a single mother on welfare, your only child is still wild and now dying. Your last chance of saving your baby is to convince the hospital to keep him as an inpatient so he can remain clean and his worsening heart failure under control until he qualifies for a transplant. You cannot let them give up on him.

Clinician: You are seeing this patient after his positive drug test and worsening heart failure have been confirmed. No center will transplant him, but he is otherwise healthy. The odds of him remaining drug free and alive long enough to qualify for transplant are slim. He will be discharged soon, essentially to go home to die. He does not qualify for hospice. The system has nothing to offer. You feel helpless. This is not why you went into medicine.

Instructor Notes: This case is an example of several different cultures unable to find common ground (Chapter 9). The patient is black, immature, afraid, and seriously ill. The mother is from a generation that does not question authority. She is unable to advocate for her only son. The Clinician is white, frustrated, and saddened by the situation. Appropriate referrals, particularly Social Services, hospice, and religious leaders, can bridge the gap when standard communication cannot.

Role Play 5: Breadwinner

The Setup: The patient is a 37-year-old poorly controlled diabetic with peripheral neuropathy, chronic low back pain, and left lower leg weakness from a previous injury. On Medicaid and other forms of social assistance, she has been hospitalized for several days. She has uncontrolled diabetes, significant impairment of Activities of Daily Living, urinary incontinence, and peripheral neuropathy. The workup of this sudden decline is inconclusive. There is no specific, correctable finding. Physical therapy has resulted in limited improvement and her Medicaid-approved hospital days are gone. Since she is unable to self-care, transfer from wheelchair to bed, or use a walker, she will need nursing home placement. The Patient appears to understand and accept the discharge plan. Yet, every morning there is a new complaint that requires workup.

Patient: You are the 37-year-old caregiver of your father who had a stroke 3 years ago. He's too weak to care for himself or work but has not applied for social assistance. He lives with you and your daughter and her two small children in your government-assisted housing. The entire family is dependent upon your income and housing. Despite your worsening condition, you help with childcare and your father while your daughter looks for work and goes to school, training to become a beautician. If you go to the nursing home, your family will be out on the street in days. They will lose not only housing but also all income. You are physically incapable of caring for yourself, much less the rest of your Family. Your only solution is to remain in the hospital, by whatever means necessary.

Clinician: You are able to improve the diabetic control of your patient, but the rest of the case has been one series of frustrations after another. As soon as one issue is addressed, another complication arises. The peripheral neuropathy and lower extremity weakness are not improving. The patient's overall condition appears to be as stable as it is ever going to be. Administration wants you to discharge the patient. But you can't help thinking there's something you're missing. You haven't seen a family member visit since the patient was admitted. A social worker will be joining everyone in a minute.

The Daughter: You are a 22-year-old daughter with two young children. You've always lived at home and depend upon your mother for help with your childcare needs. School is hard and the children demand a lot of your time. There's barely enough time to get everything done. You are scared and unsure of what to do. You can barely keep the kids in line, and now you're responsible for your grandfather, too. You're becoming overwhelmed and need your mother back home.

Social Worker: You are on your fifth case today, and it's not even 10 am! Through your earlier conversation with the daughter, you suspect that the family's situation is dependent on the patient's income. You are desperately searching for resources, but your state is limited by multiple restrictions.

Family and child services determine what you can offer. Once you've completed this task, you can join the family meeting and describe the solution you've found and convince the family this will work. The patient will enter the nursing home. The daughter, her children, and grandfather will file for Medicaid and housing with your help.

Instructor Notes: This case illustrates the value of multidisciplinary team approach with clear communication (Chapter 12). When cases are puzzling, team members provide critical input and resolution. Frequently, team members do not read the interdisciplinary notes. Face-to-face encounters, even informally, can make a huge difference in care. As soon as her Family's needs are recognized and met, the patient stabilizes and enters the nursing home without further complaint.

Role Play 6: Peer to Peer

The Setup: The local indigent healthcare clinic has an MD and PA team running all hospitalized patients. The team works efficiently and seamlessly to ensure high quality care. Most of the time, the team is single minded. Naturally, disagreements occur.

MD: A classically trained doctor specializing in Internal Medicine, you are very good at your job. With a great working relationship with your PA, you rarely countermand any order. You have the classic training of not accepting defeat with terminal patients. Due to this subconscious distaste, you avoid EOL conversations. Hospice is only for a patient in the active dying phase, transition.

PA: Working as part of this hospital team has been a dream job – especially when you are with your favorite MD. When a patient has less than 6 months to live, you want to order hospice. Conversely, your MD wants to wait until the patient is in transition. You've explained that the service can offer so much more to both Patient and Family, if the consult is done in a timely manner. He insists that it is not needed until the Patient is actively dying.

Today, you've decided to order hospice on a patient who is ready for discharge. He has poorly controlled diabetes, heart failure, and atherosclerotic disease resulting in multiple pin strokes. The patient is on maximal medical therapy and not a candidate for additional interventions. Because of his indigent status and erratic medical course, you want the additional home support hospice can give him. You know the order is going to create a discussion, but you are convinced that hospice is what's best for the patient.

Instructor Notes: Peer-to-peer disagreements occur frequently in medicine. The clear, designated hierarchy discourages opposing views and different perspectives. Timing of discussion is critical. Use of the "Four C's©" keeps emotions and preconceived notions in check (Chapter 12).

Role Play 7: Stop or Go

Setup: The patient was diagnosed with medulloblastoma, a brain tumor spanning both hemispheres. Initial diagnosis was late in childhood, at the age of 12. Therapy included a complex surgery with a difficult recovery. The patient received the maximum dose of radiation when the tumor recurred at the age of 14. Chemotherapy has slowed progression but not halted tumor growth. The patient is now 15 years of age and is frail and fatigued.

Patient: Your entire adolescence has been spent in and out of a hospital. You can't seem to beat this damned tumor. Mom and Dad do their best, as they deal with the continued surgeries, treatments, and recovery. "Normal life" has shrunk to minutes in a week. You still haven't had your first date, first kiss, nothing. In between being mad about it all, you're getting tired. Tired of being sick, tired of fighting, tired of telling Mom and Dad you're okay. Tired of the lying, because you aren't okay.

You are alone when your Clinician walks into the exam room. When he/she asks how you are doing, you tell the truth. You want to stop all treatment. You are done.

Parents: You've done everything – tried it all, spared no expense, and your only child is still sick. You do what you can to make life as "normal as possible." There must be some medical miracle to turn the tide. Every day with him/her is a win against this disease. You must keep fighting.

Clinician: This patient grew up in your care. This young person is your Family. The prognosis is dismal. You see the weariness in the patient's eyes. They want to discontinue treatment. You realize the patient is protecting his/her parents. The adolescent's emotions are masked when the parents walk into the room. Your patient needs support in telling Mom and Dad it's time to stop.

Instructor's notes: This is a medical, bioethical, and legal case. Assuming that they will act in the best interest of the child, parents are granted full, legal authority to decide medical care. Over the years, courts have begun to recognize that children under the age of 18 can show maturity and competence in making their choices. Courts recognize that children of serious, long-term illnesses mature more rapidly than their peers. Although a minor, the Patient's rights and preferences need to be considered in any significant decision.

Giving the Patient a voice in this type of situation is difficult and necessary. *Voicing My Choices* is a tool for adolescents and young adults to express their preferences (see Chapter 11). State laws vary on when a child can have a role in deciding their care choices. An ethics consult should be obtained to navigate the ethical and legal waters.

APPENDIX B

Tools for Clinicians

1

Spiritual Assessment Questions from the Joint Commission on Accreditation of Healthcare Organizations (A template for Spiritual Assessment: A review of the JCAHO requirements and guidelines (2004) found at jointcommission. org/standards/standard-faq/critical-access-hospital/provision-of-care-treatment-and-+services-pc/000001669/)

2

Personal Loss History: One way to become more self-aware and healthy in processing loss is by developing a personal loss history. Listed in the following are questions to help explore and define personal loss.

1 The first death I can remember was the death of:
2 I was age:
3 The feelings I remember I had at the time were:
4 The first funeral (wake or other ritual services) I ever attended was for:
5 I was age:
6 The thing I most remember about that experience is:
7 My most recent loss by death was (person, time, circumstances):
8 I coped with this loss by:
9 The most difficult death for me was the death of:
10 It was difficult because:
11 Of all the important people in my life who are now living, the most difficult death for me would be the death of:
12 It would be difficult because:
13 My primary style of coping with loss is:

14 I know my own grief is resolved when:

15 It is appropriate for me to share my own experiences of grief with a patient when:

3

Harvard Implicit Bias Testing: The following link has the free test and assessment: https://implicit.harvard.edu/implicit/takeatest.html

4

Behaviors associated with chemical dependency. (Quinlan, D. (1995) The Impaired anesthesia provider: the manager's role. *AANA Journal*. 63(6))

1 Isolates and withdraws from peers

2 Increasing or unexplained tardiness or absenteeism

3 Unwillingness or inability to communicate feelings

4 Increasing mood lability with frequent unexplained anger, overreacts to criticism

5 Frequent illness or physical complaints

6 Dishonesty, often over trivial or unimportant matters

7 Increasing difficulty with peers, supervisors, and authority

8 Frequent home crises – family illness and situational problems

9 Gradual and subtle deterioration of routine work performance

10 Inappropriate dress and hygiene

11 Disappears and disappoints patients and peers during work

12 Evidence of alcohol or drug use, odor of alcohol on breath, heavy perfume or mouthwash

13 Tremors, "Monday morning shakes"

14 Waits until alone to open narcotics cabinet

15 Wears long sleeves all the time

16 Consistently signs out more narcotics than peers

17 Forgetful, unpredictable

18 Frequent bathroom breaks

19 Making preoperative rounds or visits at unusual hours

20 Showing up on time off and around departmental drug supply

21 Intoxicated at social functions

22 Makes inappropriate choice or amount of drug

23 Makes use of infrequently used drugs

5

Enabling behaviors of colleagues of impaired providers. (Quinlan, D. (1995) The Impaired anesthesia provider: the manager's role. *AANA Journal*. 63(6))

1 Accepting the impaired provider's (IP) responsibilities and duties

2 Repressing own feelings, reacting defensively

3   Feeling superior, self-righteous about IP
4   Avoiding, withdrawing from situation
5   Believing they can fix the IP's behavior
6   Moralizing, judging, blaming the IP for own bad feelings
7   Denying or minimizing the severity of the problem
8   Protecting the IP from consequences of their usage by lying, covering, and protecting the IP's image
9   Believing the IP can control their usage and behavior
10 Accepting the IP's rationalizations, excuses, and promises
11 Reasoning with and enduring the IP's behaviors
12 Confronting with generalities, opinions, and judgments
13 Expressing vague, general demands for change that promote denial
14 Failing to follow through on ultimatums

6

Professional Quality of Life Scale (ProQoL) (Adapted from Stamm, B. H. (2016, January). The secondary effects of helping others: A comprehensive bibliography of 2,017 scholarly publications using the terms compassion fatigue, compassion satisfaction, secondary traumatic stress, vicarious traumatization, vicarious transformation, and ProQOL. www.proqol.org.)

When you care for people, you have direct contact with their lives. As you may have found, your compassion for those you care for can affect you in positive and negative ways. The following are some questions about your experiences, both positive and negative as a caregiver. Consider each of the following questions about you and your current work situation. Select the number that honestly reflects how frequently you experienced these things in the last *30 days*.

1 = Never,   2 = Rarely,   3 = Sometimes,   4 = Often,   5 = Very Often

_____   1   I am happy.
_____   2   I am preoccupied with more than one patient.
_____   3   I get satisfaction from being able to care for patients.
_____   4   I feel connected to others.
_____   5   I jump or am startled by unexpected sounds.
_____   6   I feel invigorated after working with patients.
_____   7   I find it difficult to separate my personal life from my life as a caregiver.
_____   8   I am not as productive at work because I am losing sleep over the traumatic experiences of a patient.
_____   9   I think I might have been affected by the traumatic stress of patients.
_____ 10   I feel trapped by my job as a caregiver.
_____ 11   Because of my caregiving, I have felt "on edge" about various things.
_____ 12   I like my work as a clinician.
_____ 13   I feel depressed because of the traumatic experiences of the patients I treat.
_____ 14   I feel as though I am experiencing the trauma of someone I have treated.
_____ 15   I have beliefs that sustain me.
_____ 16   I am pleased with how I am able to keep up with medical techniques and protocols.
_____ 17   I am the person I always wanted to be.
_____ 18   My work makes me feel satisfied.
_____ 19   I feel worn out because of my work as a clinician.
_____ 20   I have happy thoughts and feelings about my patients and how I could help them.
_____ 21   I feel overwhelmed because my caseload seems endless.
_____ 22   I believe I can make a difference through my work.

_____ 23 I avoid certain activities or situations because they remind me of frightening experiences of patients I've served.

_____ 24 I am proud of what I do to help patients.

_____ 25 As a result of my caregiving, I have intrusive, frightening thoughts.

_____ 26 I feel "bogged down" by the system.

_____ 27 I have thoughts that I am a "success" as a clinician.

_____ 28 I can't recall important parts of my work with trauma victims.

_____ 29 I am a very caring person.

_____ 30 I am happy that I chose to do this work.

Scoring your test. In this section, you will score the test, so you understand the interpretation for yourself. To find your score on each section, total the questions listed on the left then find your score on the table on the right of the section.

TABLE B6.A Compassion Satisfaction Scale

Copy your rating on each of these questions onto this table and add them up. When you have added them up, you can find your score on the table to the right.

3. _____
6. _____
12. _____
16. _____
18. _____
20. _____
22. _____
24. _____
27. _____
30. _____
Total: _____

The Sum of My Compassion Satisfaction Questions Is	So My Score Equals	My Compassion Satisfaction Level Is
22 or less	43 or less	Low
Between 23 and 41	Around 50	Average
41 or more	57 or more	High

TABLE B6.B Burnout Scale

On the burnout scale, you will need to take an extra step. Starred items are "reverse scored." If you scored the item 1, write a 5 beside it. These questions are asked in a positive way though they tell more in the negative form. For example, question 1. "I am happy" tells us more about the effects of helping when you are *not* happy so you reverse the score.

★1. _____ = _____
★4. _____ = _____
8. _____
10. _____
★15. _____ = _____
★17. _____ = _____

You Wrote	Change to
	5
2	4
3	3
4	2
5	1

19. _____
21. _____
26. _____
★29 _____ = _____
Total: _____

TABLE B6.C Burnout Scale Results

The Sum of Burnout Questions Is	So My Score Equals	And My Burnout Level Is
22 or less	43 or less	Low
Between 23 and 41	Around 50	Average
42 or more	57 or more	High

TABLE B6.D Secondary Traumatic Stress Scale

Just like you did on Compassion Satisfaction, copy your rating on each of these questions onto this table and add them up. When you have added them up, your score can be found on the table to the right.

2. _____
5. _____
7. _____
9. _____
11. _____
13. _____
14. _____
23. _____
25. _____
28. _____
Total: _____

The Sum of My Secondary Trauma Questions Is	So My Score Equals	And My Secondary Traumatic Stress Level Is
22 or less	43 or less	Low
Between 23 and 41	Around 50	Average
42 or more	57 or more	High

	Never	Rarely	Occasionally	Often	Very Often
1 I feel emotionally numb	1	2	3	4	5
2 My heart starts pounding when I think about my work	1	2	3	4	5
3 It seems like I was reliving my patient's trauma	1	2	3	4	5
4 I have trouble sleeping	1	2	3	4	5
5 I feel discouraged about the future	1	2	3	4	5
6 Reminders of my work are upsetting	1	2	3	4	5
7 I have little interest in being around others	1	2	3	4	5
8 I feel jumpy	1	2	3	4	5
9 I am less active than usual	1	2	3	4	5
10 I think about my work when I don't intend to	1	2	3	4	5
11 I have trouble concentrating	1	2	3	4	5
12 I avoid people, places, or things that remind me of work	1	2	3	4	5

	Never	Rarely	Occasionally	Often	Very Often
13 I have disturbing dreams about work	1	2	3	4	5
14 I want to avoid some patients	1	2	3	4	5
15 I am easily annoyed	1	2	3	4	5
16 I expect something bad to happen	1	2	3	4	5
17 I notice gaps in my memory about cases	1	2	3	4	5

7

TABLE B7 Secondary Traumatic Stress Scale, short form (Bride, B. E., Robinson, M. R, Yegidis, B, and Figley, C. R. (2004) Development and validation of the Secondary Traumatic Stress Scale. *Research on Social Work Practice*, *14*, 27–35)

Read each statement, then indicate how frequently the statement was true for you in the past seven (7) days.

Scoring:

Intrusion Scale (add items 2, 3, 6, 10, 13) _____
Avoidance Scale (add items 1, 5, 7, 9, 12, 14, 17) _____
Arousal Scale (add items 4, 8, 11, 15, 16) _____
Total (add all scales)   _____

8

Maslach Burnout Inventory can be reached through the following link: Mindgarden.com/117-maslach-burnout-inventory-mbi.

9

TABLE B8 Event Scale-6: Impact of Event Scale (IES) Screening Tool for Post-Traumatic Stress Disorder (PTSD). The Test Consists of Three Specific Indicators Regarding a Traumatic Event That May Result in PTSD: Intrusion (I), Avoidance (A), and Hyperarousal (H) (Hosey, M., Leoutsakos, J. M., Li, X., Dinglas, V., Bienvenu, J., Parker, A., Hopkins, R., Needham, D., & Neufeld, K. (2019). Screening for posttraumatic stress disorder in ARDS survivors: Validation of the Impact of Event Scale (IES-6). *Critical Care 23*(1):276)

IES Statement	Item
I thought about it when I didn't mean to	I
I felt watchful or on-guard	H
Other things kept making me think about it	I
I was aware that I still have feelings about it, but I didn't deal with them	A
I try not to think about it	A
I had trouble concentrating	H

10

Five Wishes Review the *Five Wishes Advance Directives* sample offered by Aging With Dignity found at the following site: fivewishes.org/doc/default-source/Samples/five-wishes-sample.pdf

The form can be ordered through the following site: fivewishes.org

11

POLST: Using the following links, review the POLST guide and form. Most states have their own forms and terms for these portable order sets. You are responsible for determining which can be used in your area and facility.

National POLST Form Guide: https://polst.org/form-guide-pdf
National POLST Form: https://polst.org/national-polst-form-pdf

12

American Medical Association Futility Code can be found at the following link (American Medical Association. (2016). E-2.037 Medical futility in end-of-life care. *AMA code of ethics*. Retrieved 9/15/21, from www.ama-assn.org/ama/pub/category/8390.html)

INDEX

Printed in the United States
by Baker & Taylor Publisher Services

Printed in the United States
by Baker & Taylor Publisher Services